Clinical Judgment for Nursing Students:

A Complete Guide

Mastering the NCSBN Clinical Judgment Model

for Nursing School and the NCLEX

Dr. David P. Zapencki, DNP, MSN/Ed, CNE, CCRN

Professional Development Publishing

ISBN (Paperback): 978-1-971135-02-1
ISBN (eBook): 978-1-971135-03-8

Published by Professional Development Publishing.

Preface

Clinical judgment is the cornerstone of safe, effective nursing practice. Every assessment you make, every intervention you choose, every outcome you evaluate represents a direct impact on patient safety. There is no room for error—and yet, clinical judgment remains one of the most challenging skills for nursing students to master.

This workbook was written with one goal in mind: to transform clinical decision-making from a source of anxiety into a source of confidence.

The chapters that follow take a deliberate, scaffolded approach built around the NCSBN Clinical Judgment Measurement Model. We begin with foundational concepts—understanding the six cognitive skills that form the bedrock of every clinical decision. From there, we progress through increasingly complex scenarios across medical-surgical, pediatric, maternal-newborn, mental health, and critical care nursing. Each chapter builds on the last, reinforcing core skills while introducing new complexity.

What sets this text apart is its emphasis on thinking like a nurse. Nursing is not about memorizing algorithms in isolation; it is about applying clinical reasoning in real patient care scenarios. That is why you will find not only practice problems but also multi-step clinical scenarios, cue recognition exercises, and the kind of critical thinking questions you will encounter on the NCLEX and in your nursing career.

To the student reading this: clinical judgment can be learned. It requires practice, patience, and a willingness to work through problems step by step. Do not skip ahead. Do not rush. Master each chapter before moving to the next. Use the practice scenarios. Check your work against the answer key. Understand not just *what* the answer is, but *why*.

Your future patients are counting on your judgment. This book will help you develop the skills and confidence to deliver safe, thoughtful nursing care every time.

Welcome to your journey toward mastery.

Dr. David P. Zapencki

List of Figures

CHAPTER 1

Foundations of Clinical Judgment

1.1 Overview: Why Clinical Judgment Matters

Clinical judgment is the process nurses use to make decisions about patient care. It involves observing, interpreting, responding, and reflecting on patient data to provide safe and effective nursing care. Unlike simple task completion, clinical judgment requires nurses to think critically about complex, often ambiguous situations where there may not be a single "right" answer.

According to the National Council of State Boards of Nursing (NCSBN), clinical judgment can be understood as the conclusion a nurse reaches after applying critical thinking and decision-making processes to a clinical situation (NCSBN, 2018). In practice, this means taking the knowledge you've learned in nursing school and applying it to real patients with real problems in real time.

Clinical judgment is not an innate talent that some nurses possess and others lack. It is a skill that can be learned, practiced, and refined over time. The purpose of this workbook is to help you develop that skill systematically, using the same framework that the NCLEX now uses to measure clinical judgment.

Benefits for Nursing Students

For nursing students, developing strong clinical judgment skills offers several important advantages:

Bridges the theory-practice gap. One of the most challenging aspects of nursing education is translating what you learn in the classroom to what you encounter in clinical settings. Patients don't present with textbook symptoms, and real-world situations are messy and unpredictable. Clinical judgment provides a systematic framework for applying your theoretical knowledge to actual patient care situations, helping you connect the dots between what you've memorized and what you're seeing at the bedside.

Prepares you for the NCLEX. The NCLEX-RN underwent a significant change in April 2023 with the introduction of Next Generation NCLEX (NGN) items specifically designed to measure clinical judgment. These new question types—including extended multiple response, highlight, matrix, and drag-and-drop items—now comprise a substantial portion of the exam. Students who understand the clinical judgment framework and have practiced applying it to patient scenarios are better prepared to succeed on these challenging new item types.

Reduces anxiety in clinical settings. Clinical rotations can be overwhelming, especially early in your nursing education. When you're faced with a patient whose condition is changing, it's easy to freeze or panic. Having a mental framework for working through clinical problems—recognizing cues, analyzing them, prioritizing, and acting—gives you a roadmap to follow even when you feel uncertain. This structured approach can significantly reduce anxiety and build confidence.

Builds transferable thinking skills. The cognitive skills you develop through clinical judgment practice don't just apply to one specialty or one type of patient. Whether you're caring for a postoperative adult, a pediatric patient with asthma, or a laboring mother, the same fundamental thinking process applies. Mastering this framework now will serve you throughout your entire nursing career, regardless of where you practice.

Develops professional identity. Nurses are not simply task-completers who follow physician orders. Nursing is an autonomous profession with its own body of knowledge and scope of practice. Clinical judgment is at the heart of what makes nursing a profession. Developing these skills helps you begin to think of yourself as a clinical decision-maker, not just a caregiver who performs procedures.

Benefits for Practicing Nurses

Strong clinical judgment skills continue to benefit nurses throughout their careers:

Improves patient outcomes. Research consistently demonstrates that nurses with strong clinical judgment skills achieve better patient outcomes. They recognize deterioration earlier, intervene more appropriately, and prevent complications before they become life-threatening. In an era of increasing patient acuity and complexity, the ability to make sound clinical decisions quickly is more important than ever.

Increases efficiency. Nurses today care for more patients with higher acuity levels than ever before. Strong clinical judgment allows you to quickly identify what matters most, prioritize your actions, and allocate your time effectively. Rather than treating every piece of data as equally important, you learn to filter, focus, and act decisively.

Reduces errors and near-misses. Many medical errors result from failures in clinical reasoning—missing important cues, drawing incorrect conclusions, or failing to act on concerning findings. Systematic clinical judgment reduces the risk of these cognitive errors by ensuring you consider all relevant data, generate appropriate hypotheses, and evaluate the effectiveness of your interventions.

Supports professional autonomy. Nurses with strong clinical judgment are better able to advocate for their patients, communicate effectively with physicians and other team members, and practice to the full extent of their scope. They can articulate not just what they observed, but what it means and what should be done about it.

Enhances job satisfaction. Feeling competent and confident in your clinical decision-making contributes significantly to job satisfaction. Nurses who trust their own judgment experience less burnout, feel more engaged in their work, and are more likely to remain in the profession long-term.

Supports career advancement. Clinical judgment is a foundational competency for advanced practice roles, leadership positions, and specialty certifications. Nurses who demonstrate strong clinical reasoning are often identified as leaders and selected for advancement opportunities.

Benefits for Patients

Ultimately, the most important beneficiaries of strong clinical judgment are the patients we serve:

Safer care. Patients are safer when their nurses can recognize early warning signs of deterioration, interpret assessment findings accurately, and intervene before conditions become critical. Clinical judgment is quite literally a matter of life and death. Studies have shown that failure to rescue—the inability to recognize and respond to patient deterioration—is a leading cause of preventable hospital deaths.

Earlier intervention. The nurse is often the first healthcare provider to notice that something is wrong. A patient's subtle change in mental status, a slight increase in respiratory rate, or a vague complaint of not feeling right may be the earliest indicators of a serious problem. Nurses with strong clinical judgment recognize these cues and act on them before the situation deteriorates.

More individualized care. Clinical judgment involves considering not just the patient's diagnosis, but their unique circumstances, preferences, and responses to treatment. This leads to more personalized, patient-centered care that respects individual differences and promotes better engagement in the treatment plan.

Better communication. Nurses with strong clinical judgment can explain what is happening, why certain interventions are necessary, and what to expect. This clear communication helps patients and families understand their care, reduces anxiety, and promotes trust in the healthcare team.

Reduced complications and shorter hospital stays. When problems are identified early and addressed appropriately, patients experience fewer complications, recover faster, and often have shorter hospital stays. This benefits not only the individual patient but also the healthcare system as a whole.

Increased confidence in care. Patients can sense when their nurse is competent and confident. When patients trust that their nurse knows what to look for, understands what the findings mean, and will take appropriate action, they feel safer and more secure in their care.

The Bottom Line

Clinical judgment is not optional—it is essential. It is the core competency that separates a truly effective nurse from one who simply completes tasks. The good news is that clinical judgment can be developed through deliberate practice, and that is exactly what this workbook is designed to help you do.

In the chapters that follow, you will learn a systematic approach to clinical decision-making based on the NCSBN Clinical Judgment Measurement Model. You will practice recognizing relevant cues, analyzing what they mean, prioritizing your hypotheses, generating appropriate solutions, taking action, and evaluating outcomes. With each case study and practice problem, your clinical judgment skills will grow stronger.

Your patients deserve a nurse who can think critically, act decisively, and adapt to changing situations. This workbook will help you become that nurse.

1.2 The NCSBN Clinical Judgment Measurement Model

The NCSBN Clinical Judgment Measurement Model (NCJMM) provides a framework for understanding how nurses make clinical decisions. Developed by the National Council of State Boards of Nursing and first published in 2018, this model represents years of research into how nurses think, reason, and act in clinical situations (Dickison, Haerling, & Lasater, 2019). Understanding this model is essential not only for NCLEX preparation but also for developing the systematic thinking skills you will use throughout your nursing career.

Note: *The NCJMM, including its three-layer structure and six cognitive skills (Recognize Cues, Analyze Cues, Prioritize Hypotheses, Generate Solutions, Take Action, and Evaluate Outcomes), is the intellectual property of NCSBN. The framework is presented here for educational purposes to help students understand and apply the model in their clinical practice and NCLEX preparation.*

History and Development

The NCJMM emerged from a recognition that traditional nursing education and testing methods did not adequately capture how nurses actually make decisions in practice. While nurses have always used clinical judgment, there was no standardized framework for teaching, measuring, or evaluating this essential competency.

In 2013, NCSBN began a multi-year research initiative to develop a model that would accurately represent clinical judgment in nursing practice. Researchers reviewed existing literature on clinical reasoning—including Christine Tanner's influential work on thinking like a nurse (Tanner, 2006)—conducted focus groups with practicing nurses, and analyzed real-world clinical scenarios to understand the cognitive processes nurses use when making decisions.

The resulting model was published by NCSBN in 2018 and became the foundation for the Next Generation NCLEX (NGN), which launched in April 2023 (NCSBN, 2023). The NGN introduced new item types specifically designed to measure clinical judgment, making the NCJMM directly relevant to every nursing student preparing for licensure.

Relationship to the Nursing Process

If you are already familiar with the traditional nursing process (Assessment, Diagnosis, Planning, Implementation, Evaluation), you may notice similarities to the clinical judgment model. This is intentional—the NCJMM builds upon and refines the nursing process rather than replacing it. The key difference is that the clinical judgment model breaks down the Diagnosis step into two distinct cognitive skills: Analyze Cues and Prioritize Hypotheses. This separation emphasizes the critical thinking required to interpret data and determine which problems are most urgent.

Figure 1.1: Nursing Process vs. Clinical Judgment Model

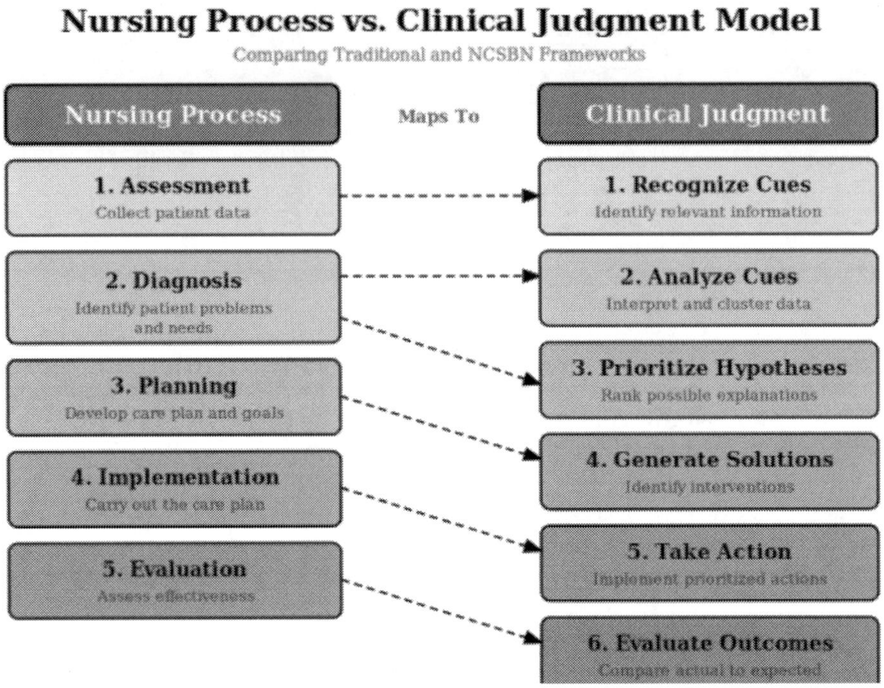

The Clinical Judgment Model expands the Diagnosis step into two distinct cognitive skills.

The Three Layers of the Model

The NCJMM is structured as three concentric layers, each representing different factors that influence clinical judgment. Understanding these layers helps you appreciate that clinical judgment doesn't happen in a vacuum—it is shaped by the patient's needs, your own characteristics as a nurse, and the cognitive skills you apply.

Layer 0: Client Needs. At the center of the model is the patient. Everything in clinical judgment begins with and returns to the patient's needs. This layer encompasses the patient's health status, presenting problems, medical history, psychosocial factors, and care environment. The patient's needs create the context for all clinical decision-making. A patient experiencing chest pain in the emergency department presents different clinical judgment challenges than a patient with the same complaint in a long-term care facility. The client's unique circumstances—their age, comorbidities, support system, preferences, and goals—all influence how you interpret data and make decisions.

Layer 1: Environmental and Individual Factors. The second layer represents variables that affect the nurse's ability to make clinical judgments. These factors don't change the "right" answer, but they influence how easily or quickly a nurse can arrive at that answer.

> *Environmental factors* include time pressure, available resources, task complexity, staffing levels, interruptions, and the overall care environment. A nurse working in a chaotic, understaffed unit faces different challenges than one working in a well-resourced setting with adequate support.

> *Individual factors* include the nurse's knowledge, experience, specialty background, and prior exposure to similar situations. A novice nurse and an experienced ICU nurse may both arrive at the correct clinical judgment, but the path they take—and the speed with which they arrive—will differ based on their individual characteristics.

Layer 2: The Six Cognitive Skills. The outermost layer contains the six cognitive skills that form the core of clinical judgment: Recognize Cues, Analyze Cues, Prioritize Hypotheses, Generate Solutions, Take Action, and Evaluate Outcomes. These are the mental processes nurses use to move from recognizing a problem to resolving it. Each skill builds on the previous one, though in practice, nurses often move fluidly between them rather than following a strict linear sequence.

How the Layers Interact

The three layers of the NCJMM do not operate independently—they interact continuously throughout the clinical judgment process. Consider this example:

> A 72-year-old patient with heart failure (Layer 0: client needs) presents with increasing shortness of breath. A new graduate nurse working a busy night shift with five other patients (Layer 1: environmental and individual factors) must recognize that the patient's respiratory rate has increased (Recognize Cues), connect this finding to the patient's cardiac history and assess for other signs of fluid overload (Analyze Cues), determine whether this represents worsening heart failure or a new problem like pneumonia (Prioritize Hypotheses), identify appropriate interventions (Generate Solutions), implement the most urgent actions first (Take Action), and reassess to determine if the patient is improving (Evaluate Outcomes).

In this scenario, the patient's underlying condition shapes what cues are relevant. The nurse's experience level and workload affect how quickly she can process the information. And the six cognitive skills provide the framework for working through the problem systematically.

The Iterative Nature of Clinical Judgment

While the six cognitive skills are often presented in a linear sequence, real-world clinical judgment is rarely so straightforward. The process is iterative, meaning you may cycle through the skills multiple times as a situation evolves.

For example, after taking action and evaluating outcomes, you may recognize new cues that require you to start the process again. Or while generating solutions, you may realize you need to gather more data, sending you back to recognizing and analyzing cues. This back-and-forth movement is normal and reflects the dynamic nature of patient care.

The model also acknowledges that experienced nurses often compress or combine steps. An ICU nurse who has cared for hundreds of patients with sepsis may recognize a pattern almost instantly and move directly to action, while a novice nurse needs to work through each step deliberately. Both approaches can lead to good clinical judgment—the difference is in the speed and automaticity of the process.

Why This Model Matters

The NCJMM matters for several important reasons:

It provides a common language. By defining clinical judgment in specific, measurable terms, the model gives nurses, educators, and researchers a shared vocabulary for discussing clinical reasoning. When your instructor asks you to "analyze cues," you know exactly what cognitive process they're referring to.

It makes thinking visible. Clinical judgment often happens invisibly, inside a nurse's head. The NCJMM breaks down this "black box" into distinct, teachable components. This makes it possible to identify where your clinical reasoning is strong and where it needs development.

It supports deliberate practice. Because the model identifies specific cognitive skills, you can practice each one individually. Rather than hoping your clinical judgment will somehow improve with experience, you can target your practice to develop specific skills.

It aligns education with practice. The NCJMM was developed from research on how nurses actually think in clinical settings. This means that practicing with this model prepares you for real-world nursing, not just for passing an exam.

It forms the basis for NCLEX testing. The Next Generation NCLEX uses the NCJMM as its framework for clinical judgment questions. Understanding the model helps you understand what these questions are really asking and how to approach them systematically.

Applying the Model in This Workbook

Throughout this workbook, you will use the NCJMM as your framework for working through clinical scenarios. Each case study will guide you through all six cognitive skills, helping you develop a systematic approach to clinical decision-making.

In the next section, we will examine each of the six cognitive skills in detail, exploring what each one involves and how to develop proficiency in it. Later chapters will give you extensive practice applying these skills to realistic patient scenarios across multiple nursing specialties.

As you work through this material, remember that the goal is not to memorize the model but to internalize it—to make systematic clinical reasoning so automatic that it becomes second nature. With practice, you will find yourself naturally recognizing cues, analyzing their meaning, and working through the clinical judgment process without consciously thinking about each step.

1.3 The Six Cognitive Skills

The core of the NCJMM consists of six cognitive skills that nurses use in clinical practice (NCSBN, 2018). These skills represent the mental processes that move a nurse from initial observation of a patient to effective intervention and evaluation. While presented here in sequence, remember that clinical judgment in practice is often iterative—you may cycle through these skills multiple times as a situation evolves.

Each cognitive skill builds on the previous one, creating a logical progression from data gathering to outcome evaluation. Mastering each skill individually will help you develop the integrated clinical reasoning that characterizes expert nursing practice.

Figure 1.2: Clinical Judgment Cycle

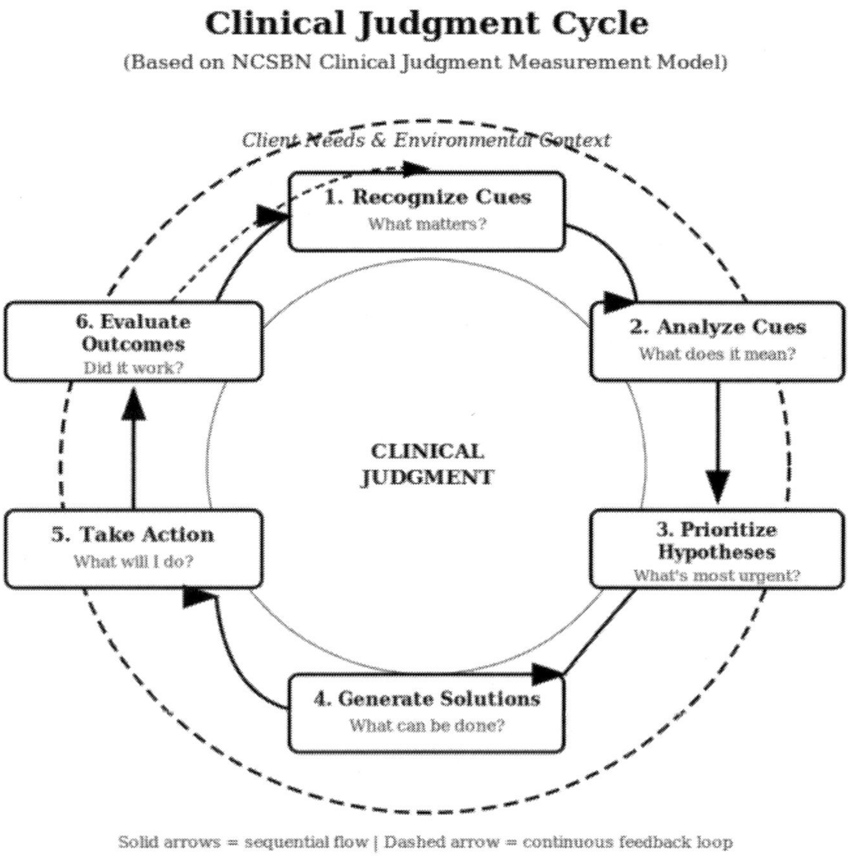

Adapted from NCSBN (2018). The process is continuous and iterative.

Recognize Cues

The first cognitive skill involves identifying relevant information from the clinical situation (NCSBN, 2018). This includes data from multiple sources: what the patient tells you (subjective data), what you observe and measure (objective data), information from the medical record, input from family members, and reports from other healthcare team members.

Recognizing cues is more than just collecting data—it requires you to filter through large amounts of information to identify what is clinically significant. In any patient encounter, you will be exposed to dozens of data points. The skill lies in determining which pieces of information matter most for this particular patient in this particular situation.

Key questions to ask yourself:

- What information stands out as abnormal or unexpected?
- What data points have changed from the patient's baseline?
- What is the patient telling me through their words, behavior, or appearance?
- What information from the chart is most relevant right now?

- What might I be missing? What haven't I assessed yet?

Novice nurses sometimes struggle with this skill because they lack the experience to know what "normal" looks like. With practice, you will develop pattern recognition that allows you to quickly spot deviations from expected findings. This workbook provides extensive practice in identifying relevant cues across a variety of clinical scenarios.

Analyze Cues

Once you have identified relevant cues, the next step is to determine what they mean (NCSBN, 2018). Analysis involves connecting individual data points to each other and to your nursing knowledge to understand the clinical picture. This is where you move from "what do I see?" to "what does it mean?"

Effective cue analysis requires you to cluster related findings together. A single abnormal vital sign might not be significant on its own, but when combined with other findings, a pattern emerges. For example, an elevated heart rate could have many causes, but when you cluster it with fever, elevated white blood cell count, and localized redness at an IV site, the pattern suggests infection.

Key questions to ask yourself:

- How do these findings relate to each other?
- What patterns or clusters do I see in the data?
- Are these findings expected or unexpected given the patient's condition?
- How do these findings compare to normal values or the patient's baseline?
- What does my nursing knowledge tell me about these findings?

Analysis also involves distinguishing between findings that are expected for a patient's condition and those that signal a problem. Some abnormalities are anticipated—for instance, mild incisional pain after surgery is expected. The skill is in recognizing when findings cross the line from expected to concerning.

Prioritize Hypotheses

Based on your analysis, you will generate possible explanations for what is happening with the patient (NCSBN, 2018). A hypothesis in this context is an educated guess about the underlying cause of the patient's signs and symptoms. Prioritizing means ranking these possibilities by both probability (what is most likely) and urgency (what is most dangerous if missed).

This skill reflects a fundamental principle in clinical reasoning: think about the worst-case scenario first. While you should consider all reasonable explanations, you must be especially vigilant for conditions that could rapidly deteriorate or become life-threatening. Even if a dangerous condition is less likely than a benign one, it may need to be ruled out first.

Key questions to ask yourself:

- What are all the possible explanations for these findings?
- Which explanation is most likely given the evidence?
- Which explanation, if true, would be most dangerous?
- What conditions must I rule out before assuming a less serious cause?
- How does the patient's history affect the likelihood of each hypothesis?

Prioritization frameworks like ABCs (Airway, Breathing, Circulation) and Maslow's Hierarchy of Needs can guide your thinking. Physiological threats take precedence over psychological ones, and immediate life threats take precedence over long-term concerns. These frameworks, long established in nursing practice, help ensure you address the most critical issues first (Alfaro-LeFevre, 2020).

Generate Solutions

With prioritized hypotheses in mind, you now identify potential interventions to address the patient's needs (NCSBN, 2018). This skill involves drawing on your nursing knowledge to determine what actions could help—including independent nursing interventions, collaborative interventions requiring physician orders, and referrals to other healthcare professionals.

Generating solutions requires you to consider multiple options, not just the first intervention that comes to mind. Different situations call for different approaches, and you must weigh the benefits, risks, and feasibility of each option. You should also anticipate potential complications and plan accordingly.

Key questions to ask yourself:

- What interventions could address the priority hypothesis?
- What does the evidence say about effective interventions for this situation?
- What resources are available to me right now?
- What are the potential risks or complications of each option?
- Who else needs to be involved in addressing this problem?

Evidence-based practice plays a crucial role in generating solutions. Your interventions should be grounded in current best evidence whenever possible. This means staying current with nursing research and clinical guidelines, and knowing how to access reliable information when you encounter unfamiliar situations (Melnyk & Fineout-Overholt, 2019).

Take Action

This skill involves implementing your chosen intervention(s) in a timely, safe, and appropriate manner (NCSBN, 2018). Taking action encompasses not only performing the intervention itself but also prioritizing when you have multiple actions to complete, delegating appropriately to other team members, and communicating effectively with patients, families, and colleagues.

Action without proper prioritization can be dangerous. When a patient has multiple needs, you must determine which actions to perform first. The same frameworks that guide hypothesis prioritization—ABCs, Maslow's Hierarchy—also guide action prioritization. Address immediate threats to life before other concerns.

Key questions to ask yourself:

- What is the most urgent action I need to take right now?
- In what order should I complete multiple actions?
- Can any of these actions be safely delegated? To whom?
- What information must I communicate, and to whom?
- What must I document about this situation and my actions?

Effective action also requires clear communication. When you need to notify a physician about a patient's changing condition, structured communication tools like SBAR (Situation, Background, Assessment,

Recommendation) help ensure you convey critical information clearly and receive appropriate orders in response (Institute for Healthcare Improvement, 2021).

Evaluate Outcomes

The final cognitive skill involves assessing whether your interventions achieved the desired effect (NCSBN, 2018). Evaluation compares actual patient outcomes to expected outcomes and determines whether the plan of care is working or needs modification. This step closes the loop in the clinical judgment process—and often opens a new loop as evaluation reveals new cues to recognize.

Evaluation must be systematic and timely. You should know what indicators to monitor, when to reassess, and what findings would indicate success or failure. If outcomes are not as expected, you return to earlier steps in the process—perhaps recognizing new cues, reanalyzing the situation, or generating alternative solutions.

Key questions to ask yourself:

- What outcome did I expect from my intervention?
- What outcome actually occurred?
- Did the patient's condition improve, stay the same, or worsen?
- If the outcome was not as expected, why might that be?
- What modifications to the plan of care are needed?

Evaluation is not a one-time event but an ongoing process. Patients' conditions change continuously, and what works at one moment may not work later. Skilled nurses maintain a constant cycle of evaluation, ready to recognize when the situation has changed and a new round of clinical judgment is needed.

Putting It All Together

In practice, these six cognitive skills work together as an integrated whole. While it is useful to study each skill separately, expert nurses do not consciously think "now I am recognizing cues, now I am analyzing cues." Instead, the process becomes fluid and often rapid, especially in familiar situations.

Research by Patricia Benner on the development of nursing expertise suggests that as nurses gain experience, their clinical judgment becomes increasingly intuitive—they often "know" something is wrong before they can articulate exactly why (Benner, 1984). This intuition is not magical; it is the result of extensive pattern recognition developed through repeated exposure to clinical situations. The six cognitive skills are still at work, but they operate below conscious awareness.

For students and novice nurses, making these cognitive skills explicit is essential for learning. By consciously working through each step, you build the mental habits that will eventually become automatic. This workbook is designed to give you extensive practice with each skill, helping you develop the clinical judgment that will serve you throughout your nursing career.

1.4 How the NCLEX Tests Clinical Judgment

In April 2023, the National Council of State Boards of Nursing launched the Next Generation NCLEX (NGN), a significant update to the nursing licensure examination that places clinical judgment at the center of candidate evaluation (NCSBN, 2023). Understanding how the NCLEX tests clinical judgment will help you prepare more effectively and approach exam questions with confidence.

The Evolution of the NCLEX

The NCLEX has always aimed to assess whether nursing graduates possess the minimum competency required for safe, entry-level practice. For decades, the exam relied primarily on traditional multiple-choice questions with four answer options. While these questions could assess knowledge and some aspects of application, they had limitations in measuring the complex, multi-step reasoning that characterizes real-world clinical judgment.

Research conducted by NCSBN identified a gap between what the exam measured and what nurses actually need to do in practice. Entry-level nurses must do more than select a correct answer from a list—they must recognize problems, analyze complex data, weigh competing priorities, and make decisions in the face of uncertainty. The NGN was designed to address this gap by introducing new item types that more authentically measure clinical judgment (Dickison et al., 2019).

Next Generation NCLEX Item Types

The NGN introduced several new item types, each designed to measure specific aspects of clinical judgment. These items often appear as part of case studies (called "unfolding case studies" or "stand-alone items") that present a clinical scenario and ask multiple questions about how you would respond. Here are the primary NGN item types you will encounter:

Extended Multiple Response (Select All That Apply). Unlike traditional select-all-that-apply questions, the NGN version may have partial credit scoring. This means you earn points for each correct selection and may lose points for incorrect selections. These items often ask you to identify relevant cues or appropriate interventions from a list of options.

Extended Drag-and-Drop. These items ask you to place options in a specific order or match items to categories. For example, you might be asked to prioritize nursing actions by dragging them into the correct sequence, or to match patient findings to the conditions they suggest.

Cloze (Drop-Down). In cloze items, you complete sentences or fill in blanks by selecting from drop-down menus. A single item might have multiple drop-downs, each requiring you to select the most appropriate word or phrase. These items often test your ability to analyze cues and prioritize hypotheses.

Enhanced Hot Spot (Highlighting). Highlighting items present you with text—often a nurse's note, a physician's order, or patient data—and ask you to highlight the portions that are relevant to a specific question. This directly measures your ability to recognize cues by filtering relevant from irrelevant information.

Matrix/Grid. Matrix items present a table where you must indicate whether each row meets certain criteria. For example, you might be asked to indicate which assessment findings are "expected" versus "requiring follow-up," or which interventions are "indicated" versus "contraindicated" for a specific patient.

Bowtie Items. Bowtie items are named for their visual appearance and test multiple cognitive skills in a single item. Typically, you are asked to identify a condition or problem in the center, with related actions or parameters on either side. These items integrate analysis, prioritization, and solution generation.

How Item Types Map to Cognitive Skills

Each NGN item type is designed to measure one or more of the six cognitive skills from the NCJMM. Understanding this mapping can help you approach each question type more strategically:

Cognitive Skill	Common Item Types
Recognize Cues	Highlighting, Extended Multiple Response
Analyze Cues	Matrix, Cloze (Drop-Down), Bowtie
Prioritize Hypotheses	Cloze (Drop-Down), Bowtie, Drag-and-Drop
Generate Solutions	Extended Multiple Response, Cloze, Matrix
Take Action	Drag-and-Drop (ordering), Matrix, Bowtie
Evaluate Outcomes	Matrix, Cloze, Extended Multiple Response

Unfolding Case Studies

One of the most significant features of the NGN is the unfolding case study. Rather than presenting isolated, unrelated questions, the NGN includes case studies that evolve over multiple phases—much like real patient care situations.

A typical unfolding case study presents an initial scenario, then provides new information as the case progresses. You might first be asked to recognize relevant cues in the admission assessment, then analyze those cues as new data becomes available, then prioritize when the patient's condition changes, and finally evaluate outcomes after interventions are implemented.

This format mirrors clinical practice, where patient situations evolve over time and require nurses to continually reassess and adjust their plans. It also means that earlier decisions can affect later questions—just as in real nursing practice, your initial assessment shapes your subsequent actions.

Scoring and Partial Credit

The NGN introduced a more nuanced scoring system than the traditional all-or-nothing approach. Many NGN items use partial credit scoring, meaning you can earn points for partially correct answers (NCSBN, 2023). This is particularly relevant for items with multiple components, such as select-all-that-apply or matrix items.

Different scoring rules may apply to different item types. Some items use "0/1" scoring (correct or incorrect), while others use "+/-" scoring (gaining points for correct selections, losing points for incorrect ones), and still others use "rationale" scoring based on how well your selections align with clinical reasoning.

The practical implication is that you should answer based on your best clinical judgment rather than gaming the system. Select all the options you believe are correct, and avoid selecting options you believe are incorrect. Trust your clinical reasoning.

Strategies for NGN Success

Preparing for the NGN requires more than memorizing content—it requires developing and practicing clinical judgment skills. Here are strategies that will help you succeed:

Read carefully and completely. NGN items often contain substantial amounts of information. Read the entire scenario before looking at the question, and re-read relevant portions as needed. Pay attention to details—a subtle change in vital signs or a seemingly minor patient complaint may be significant.

Identify what the question is really asking. Before selecting an answer, make sure you understand which cognitive skill the item is testing. Are you being asked to identify relevant data (recognize cues), determine what findings mean (analyze cues), or select the best action (take action)? The question stem usually provides clues.

Think like a nurse, not a test-taker. The NGN is designed to measure how you would actually think and act in clinical practice. Rather than looking for tricks or trying to game the test, approach each item as if you were really caring for the patient. What would you notice? What would concern you? What would you do?

Use the clinical judgment framework. When faced with a complex scenario, mentally walk through the six cognitive skills. What cues are present? What do they mean when analyzed together? What are the possible explanations, and which is most urgent? This systematic approach helps ensure you don't miss important considerations.

Practice with NGN-style items. Familiarity with the item formats will help you feel more comfortable on test day. This workbook provides extensive practice with scenarios and question types that mirror the NGN format. The more you practice applying clinical judgment systematically, the more natural it will become.

Manage your time wisely. NGN items, especially unfolding case studies, may require more time than traditional multiple-choice questions. Pace yourself accordingly, and don't spend too much time on any single item. If you're unsure, make your best judgment and move on.

The Bigger Picture

While passing the NCLEX is an important milestone, remember that the clinical judgment skills you develop will serve a purpose far beyond the exam. The NGN was designed to better predict which candidates will provide safe, effective patient care. By developing strong clinical judgment now, you are not just preparing for a test—you are preparing for a career.

Every patient you will ever care for will benefit from your ability to recognize subtle cues, analyze complex data, prioritize competing concerns, and take appropriate action. The work you put into developing these skills now will pay dividends throughout your nursing career.

1.5 Practice Problems (20)

For each scenario, identify which cognitive skill is primarily being tested.

1. A nurse reviews a patient's vital signs, lab values, and assessment findings to determine which data points require immediate attention. → Cognitive skill?

2. After gathering data, the nurse groups related findings together and identifies that several indicators point to possible fluid volume deficit. → Cognitive skill?

3. The nurse considers three possible causes for a patient's symptoms and determines that sepsis is the most urgent concern to rule out. → Cognitive skill?

4. The nurse identifies five possible interventions and selects the most appropriate based on the patient's current status and available resources. → Cognitive skill?

5. The nurse administers the prescribed medication, positions the patient appropriately, and documents the intervention. → Cognitive skill?

6. Two hours after the intervention, the nurse reassesses the patient to determine if the desired outcome was achieved. → Cognitive skill?

7. A patient's blood pressure reading is 88/52 mmHg. The nurse notes this is significantly lower than the baseline of 128/78 mmHg. → Cognitive skill?

8. The nurse notices that the patient's elevated heart rate, decreased urine output, and altered mental status all suggest inadequate tissue perfusion. → Cognitive skill?

9. The nurse decides that hypovolemic shock is more likely than cardiogenic shock based on the patient's recent surgical history. → Cognitive skill?

10. The nurse plans to initiate a fluid bolus, elevate the patient's legs, and notify the rapid response team. → Cognitive skill?

CHAPTER 2

Recognize Cues

2.1 Overview

Recognizing cues is the first cognitive skill in the NCSBN Clinical Judgment Measurement Model and serves as the foundation for all clinical decision-making (NCSBN, 2018). Before you can analyze a situation, prioritize concerns, or take action, you must first notice that something requires your attention. This chapter focuses on developing your ability to identify relevant and significant information from the wealth of data available in any clinical situation.

In clinical practice, nurses are constantly bombarded with information: vital signs, laboratory values, assessment findings, patient statements, family concerns, monitor alarms, physician orders, and observations from other healthcare team members. The challenge is not collecting data—modern healthcare generates enormous amounts of it. The challenge is determining which pieces of information matter most for this particular patient at this particular moment.

Expert nurses develop what appears to be an almost intuitive ability to notice important cues while filtering out noise. Research suggests this ability is not innate but develops through extensive clinical experience and deliberate practice (Benner, 1984). By understanding the principles behind cue recognition and practicing systematically, you can accelerate the development of this essential skill.

2.2 What Are Cues?

In the context of clinical judgment, a cue is any piece of information that provides insight into a patient's condition. Cues come from multiple sources and can be categorized in several ways. Understanding these categories helps ensure you gather comprehensive data and don't overlook important information.

Subjective vs. Objective Data

One of the most fundamental distinctions in nursing assessment is between subjective and objective data. Both types are valuable, and skilled nurses integrate them to form a complete clinical picture.

Subjective data consists of information that only the patient can provide—their symptoms, feelings, perceptions, and experiences. Examples include pain levels, nausea, anxiety, fatigue, and descriptions of symptom onset and character. Subjective data is often captured in the patient's own words and documented in quotation marks. While subjective data cannot be independently verified, it provides irreplaceable insight into the patient's experience and should never be dismissed.

Objective data consists of information that can be observed, measured, or verified by someone other than the patient. Examples include vital signs, laboratory values, physical examination findings, diagnostic test results, and observable behaviors. Objective data provides concrete, measurable evidence of the patient's physiological status.

In practice, subjective and objective data often work together. A patient's subjective report of chest pain (subjective) gains significance when combined with ECG changes and elevated troponin levels (objective). Similarly, objective findings like elevated blood pressure may prompt you to ask about subjective symptoms like headache or blurred vision.

Sources of Clinical Information

Cues can come from many sources, and thorough cue recognition requires attention to all of them:

The patient. The patient is always the primary source of information. This includes their verbal reports, nonverbal communication, behavior, and physical presentation. Pay attention not just to what patients say, but how they say it—tone of voice, facial expressions, and body language often communicate as much as words.

Physical assessment. Your systematic assessment provides crucial objective data. This includes inspection, auscultation, palpation, and percussion findings. The nursing physical assessment differs from a medical examination in its focus on functional status and response to illness, though there is significant overlap.

Vital signs and monitoring data. Temperature, pulse, respirations, blood pressure, oxygen saturation, and pain level provide immediate insight into physiological status. Continuous monitoring data from telemetry, pulse oximetry, and other devices adds real-time information about trends and changes.

Laboratory and diagnostic results. Lab values, imaging results, and other diagnostic tests provide objective data about organ function, infection, electrolyte balance, and disease processes. Understanding normal ranges and the clinical significance of abnormal values is essential for cue recognition.

Medical record and history. The patient's documented history—including past medical history, surgical history, medications, allergies, and previous hospital records—provides context for interpreting current findings. A symptom that might be concerning in one patient may be expected in another based on their history.

Family and caregivers. Family members and caregivers can provide valuable information about the patient's baseline status, recent changes, medication compliance, and home situation. This is particularly important for patients who cannot communicate effectively for themselves.

Healthcare team members. Nurses, physicians, therapists, and other team members share observations and concerns through verbal reports, written documentation, and formal handoff communication. Information from the previous shift, from consulting services, or from ancillary staff can all provide important cues.

Figure 2.1: Sources of Clinical Data

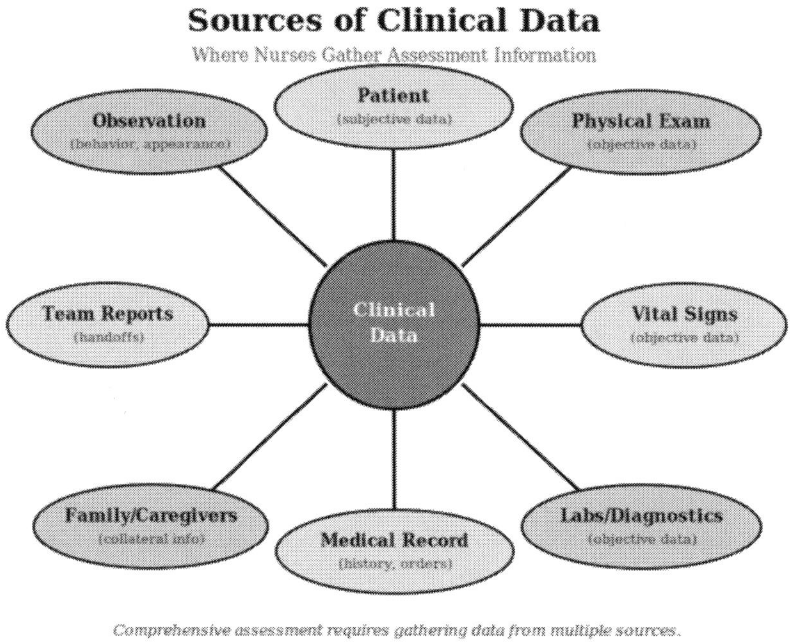

Comprehensive assessment requires gathering data from multiple sources.

2.3 Relevant vs. Irrelevant Information

Not all information is equally important. One of the most challenging aspects of cue recognition is determining which data points are clinically significant and which can be safely set aside. This skill develops with experience, but understanding the principles can help guide your thinking.

What Makes a Cue Relevant?

A cue is relevant when it provides meaningful information about the patient's current status, potential problems, or response to treatment. Several factors influence relevance:

Deviation from normal. Findings that fall outside normal physiological ranges often warrant attention. However, "normal" must be interpreted in context—what is normal for one patient may be abnormal for another. A heart rate of 90 bpm might be unremarkable for most patients but significant for someone whose baseline is 60 bpm.

Change from baseline. Changes from the patient's established baseline are often more significant than absolute values. A blood pressure that has dropped 30 mmHg from this morning's reading is concerning even if the current reading is technically within normal limits.

Relationship to the patient's condition. Cues that relate to the patient's diagnosis, treatment, or risk factors are more likely to be relevant. For a patient admitted with heart failure, weight gain and increased edema are highly relevant findings. For a patient admitted for an unrelated orthopedic procedure, the same findings might be incidental.

Potential for harm. Some cues warrant attention because they suggest a risk for serious complications, even if the current finding seems minor. A slight temperature elevation in an immunocompromised patient requires more attention than the same finding in a healthy individual.

Urgency. Cues that suggest an immediate threat to patient safety are always relevant. Airway compromise, severe chest pain, altered consciousness, or signs of hemorrhage demand immediate attention regardless of the patient's admitting diagnosis.

Filtering Out Noise

Just as important as recognizing relevant cues is the ability to filter out irrelevant information. Cognitive overload—trying to process too much information at once—impairs clinical judgment and can lead to missed cues or poor decisions (Alfaro-LeFevre, 2020). Effective nurses develop mental filters that allow them to focus on what matters.

Information is generally irrelevant when it does not relate to the patient's current clinical concerns, does not deviate meaningfully from normal or baseline values, does not suggest any risk for complications, and would not change your clinical actions regardless of its value. However, be cautious about dismissing information too quickly—what seems irrelevant initially may become significant as the clinical picture evolves.

Figure 2.2: Cue Recognition Funnel

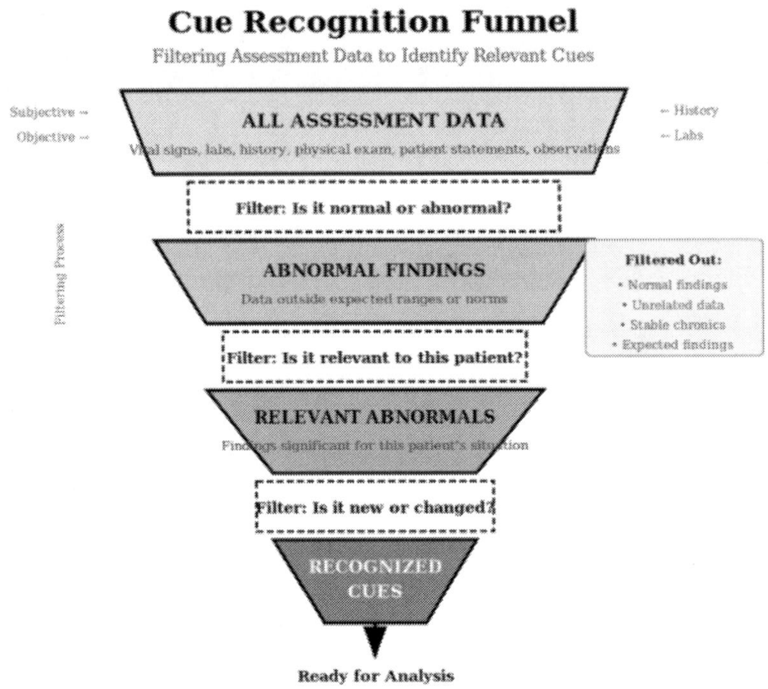

Filter data through progressive questions to identify the cues that require action.

Common Pitfalls in Cue Recognition

Several cognitive biases and errors can interfere with effective cue recognition. Being aware of these pitfalls can help you avoid them:

Anchoring bias. The tendency to focus on the first piece of information encountered and interpret subsequent information through that lens. For example, if you're told at handoff that a patient is "drug-seeking," you may be less likely to recognize cues suggesting genuine pain.

Confirmation bias. The tendency to notice information that confirms what you already believe while overlooking information that contradicts it. If you've decided a patient has a UTI, you may focus on supportive findings while missing cues that suggest a different diagnosis.

Tunnel vision. Focusing too narrowly on one problem or system while missing issues elsewhere. The patient admitted for pneumonia may also be developing a pressure injury, but if you're focused only on respiratory status, you might miss the early skin changes.

Normalization of deviance. Gradually coming to accept abnormal findings as normal because you've seen them repeatedly. A chronically understaffed unit may come to accept delayed responses to call lights as "just how it is," missing cues that patients are in distress.

Failure to recognize patterns. Missing the significance of findings that, taken together, suggest a problem. Individual vital sign changes might seem minor, but the pattern of increasing heart rate, decreasing blood pressure, and rising respiratory rate suggests shock.

2.4 Strategies for Effective Cue Recognition

While cue recognition develops naturally with clinical experience, you can accelerate your growth by employing deliberate strategies. The following approaches will help you become more systematic and effective in recognizing important clinical information.

Use a Systematic Assessment Approach

A systematic, head-to-toe or systems-based assessment ensures you don't miss important findings by forgetting to look. The specific system you use matters less than using it consistently. Whether you prefer a head-to-toe approach, a body-systems approach, or a functional health patterns framework, the key is thoroughness and consistency.

During your assessment, actively compare what you find to what you expect based on the patient's condition. Ask yourself: What should I expect to find given this patient's diagnosis and history? What am I actually finding? Where are the discrepancies? These discrepancies are often the most important cues.

Know Your Baselines

You cannot recognize change without knowing the starting point. At the beginning of your shift, establish the patient's baseline status. Review recent vital signs and trends. Read the previous shift's nursing notes. Talk with the outgoing nurse about what has been "normal" for this patient. This investment of time at the start of your shift pays dividends in your ability to recognize significant changes.

Remember that baseline varies by patient. A blood pressure of 150/90 mmHg might be elevated for most patients but represents excellent control for someone with poorly controlled hypertension. A respiratory rate of 24 might be concerning for one patient but baseline for someone with chronic lung disease.

Trust Your Instincts—But Verify

Experienced nurses often describe a "gut feeling" that something is wrong, even before they can identify specific abnormal findings. Research supports the validity of this clinical intuition—it represents pattern recognition operating below conscious awareness (Benner, 1984). If something feels wrong, take that feeling seriously.

However, intuition alone is not sufficient. When you sense something is wrong, follow up with systematic assessment to identify specific cues. What exactly is different? What findings support your concern? This verification serves two purposes: it helps you identify specific problems requiring action, and it helps you develop the explicit knowledge that will make your intuition more reliable over time.

Listen to the Patient

Patients often know when something is wrong before objective signs become apparent. Statements like "I don't feel right," "Something is different," or "I feel like something bad is going to happen" should be taken seriously. While these vague complaints may not point to a specific problem, they often represent the patient's recognition of subtle physiological changes.

This is particularly true for patients who know their own bodies well, such as those with chronic conditions. A patient with heart failure who says their breathing feels different, or a patient with diabetes who says something feels off, is often recognizing early changes before they become clinically obvious.

2.5 Clinical Application Examples

The following examples illustrate cue recognition in clinical practice. For each scenario, notice how certain findings stand out as relevant while others, though present, are less significant for the immediate clinical concern.

Example 1: Postoperative Patient

Scenario: Mr. Johnson is postoperative day 1 following abdominal surgery. During your assessment, you note: T 99.8°F, HR 88 bpm, RR 18, BP 128/76 mmHg, pain 4/10 at the incision site, bowel sounds absent, abdomen soft and non-distended, Foley catheter draining clear yellow urine 40 mL/hr, incision with staples intact and mild serous drainage on dressing.

Relevant cues: Most of these findings are expected for POD1. The low-grade temperature is common in the first 24-48 hours postoperatively due to the inflammatory response. Absent bowel sounds are expected until peristalsis returns. The pain level is controlled. These findings do not require immediate intervention.

What to monitor: Continue monitoring for return of bowel function. Watch for temperature elevation beyond 48 hours or above 101°F, which could indicate infection. Monitor incision for increased drainage, redness, or separation.

Example 2: Medical Patient with Changing Status

Scenario: Mrs. Chen, 72, was admitted yesterday with community-acquired pneumonia. At 0700, her vitals were: T 100.4°F, HR 92 bpm, RR 22, BP 118/70 mmHg, SpO2 94% on 2L NC. She was alert and conversational. At 1100, you find: T 101.8°F, HR 110 bpm, RR 28, BP 100/62 mmHg, SpO2 90% on 2L NC. She is drowsy and slow to respond to questions.

Relevant cues: This patient is deteriorating. Key cues include: rising temperature and heart rate, dropping blood pressure, increasing respiratory rate with decreasing oxygen saturation despite unchanged oxygen delivery, and altered mental status. The pattern of these changes suggests possible sepsis.

Why these matter: Each finding alone might be explained away, but the pattern of changes from her baseline 4 hours ago is significant. This patient requires immediate reassessment and likely escalation of care. The change in mental status is particularly concerning as it suggests inadequate tissue perfusion.

Example 3: Distinguishing Relevant from Irrelevant

Scenario: You are reviewing the chart for Mr. Williams, admitted for elective knee replacement scheduled for tomorrow. The chart contains extensive information including: history of hypertension controlled on lisinopril, appendectomy 30 years ago, allergy to penicillin (hives), works as an accountant, married with two adult children, cholesterol 210 mg/dL, HbA1c 5.8%, takes a daily multivitamin, has a history of mild seasonal allergies, quit smoking 20 years ago.

Most relevant for current care: Penicillin allergy (critical for antibiotic selection), hypertension and current medication (relevant for perioperative management), and smoking history (affects healing and anesthesia risk, though quit long ago).

Less immediately relevant: Occupation, family composition, multivitamin use, and seasonal allergies are less directly relevant to the surgical episode, though they contribute to understanding the patient as a whole person.

2.6 Practice Problems (20)

The following exercises will help you practice recognizing relevant cues. For each scenario, identify the most significant findings and explain why they are important.

1. A patient with heart failure has the following morning assessment: weight up 3 lbs from yesterday, 2+ pitting edema to ankles (baseline 1+), lung sounds with crackles in bases, SpO2

92% on room air (baseline 95%), patient reports sleeping in recliner because "I couldn't breathe lying flat." Which findings are most significant and why?

2. You receive a patient in handoff with the following information: 45-year-old admitted for cellulitis of left lower leg, IV antibiotics started yesterday, history of diabetes, last blood glucose 186 mg/dL, allergic to sulfa, temperature 99.2°F, patient is a vegetarian. Which pieces of information are most relevant to planning this patient's care?

3. A postpartum patient, day 1 after cesarean delivery, reports: incisional pain 6/10, fundus firm at umbilicus, moderate lochia rubra, difficulty urinating since Foley removed 2 hours ago, temperature 98.8°F. Which findings are expected, and which might require follow-up?

4. During your assessment of an elderly patient admitted for confusion, you note: oriented to name only, skin warm and dry, has not voided in 8 hours, taking hydrochlorothiazide and donepezil at home, family states "she was fine last week." What cues suggest this may be delirium rather than dementia?

5. A patient with COPD on 2L nasal cannula has the following: RR 24, SpO2 91%, using accessory muscles slightly, speaking in full sentences, states "this is my normal." Previous shift documented similar findings. How does knowing the patient's baseline affect your interpretation?

6. You are assessing a pediatric patient, age 4, admitted for asthma exacerbation. Findings include: RR 32, mild intercostal retractions, SpO2 94% on room air, audible wheezing without stethoscope, child sitting upright and appears anxious, parent states "she's had colds before but never breathed like this." Identify the relevant cues.

7. A patient admitted for alcohol withdrawal has: HR 112, BP 158/94, tremors in both hands, reports "seeing things that aren't there," diaphoretic, last drink was 36 hours ago. Which cues indicate the severity of withdrawal, and which might suggest a complication?

8. During a mental health assessment, a patient reports: "I've been thinking about ending it all," has a plan involving medications at home, gave away prized possessions last week, recently divorced, states mood is 3/10 with 10 being best. Which cues indicate highest risk?

9. A patient receiving a blood transfusion develops: temperature increase from 98.6°F to 100.2°F, reports feeling "a little itchy," no hives visible, vital signs otherwise stable, transfusion has been running for 45 minutes without previous symptoms. What cues require immediate attention?

10. An 8-hour-old newborn has the following assessment: temperature 97.8°F axillary, HR 142, RR 52 with occasional grunting, slight nasal flaring, SpO2 95% on room air, blood glucose 58 mg/dL, skin slightly mottled. Which findings are concerning for a newborn?

11. A patient 2 hours post-cardiac catheterization via right femoral approach has: right groin dressing with small amount of dried blood, right pedal pulse 2+ and equal to left, right foot warm and pink, back pain rated 4/10, reports needing to void. What cues require priority monitoring?

12. You are caring for a patient with a patient-controlled analgesia (PCA) pump for pain management. Current findings: pain 2/10, RR 10, SpO2 96%, sedation score 3 (frequently drowsy, arouses with verbal stimuli), pupils 2 mm bilaterally. Which findings concern you most?

13. A diabetic patient reports: blood glucose this morning was 72 mg/dL, feels "shaky and sweaty," ate breakfast 30 minutes ago but "couldn't finish it," took usual morning insulin dose. Identify the relevant cues and their significance.

14. A patient on day 3 of antibiotic therapy for pneumonia has: temperature now normal, WBC decreased from 15,000 to 11,000, reports feeling "much better," cough still productive but less frequent, SpO2 96% on room air. Which cues indicate improvement?

15. An elderly patient admitted from a nursing home has: sacral redness that does not blanch with pressure, is incontinent of urine, Braden Scale score of 12, serum albumin 2.8 g/dL. Which findings indicate pressure injury risk factors?

16. A patient with newly diagnosed atrial fibrillation has: HR 88 irregular, BP 134/82, no chest pain, reports occasional "fluttering" sensation, started on anticoagulation yesterday, INR today 1.2. Which cues require monitoring or follow-up?

17. A pre-operative patient scheduled for surgery in 2 hours tells you: "I'm so nervous I could throw up," has not eaten since midnight as instructed, took blood pressure medication this morning with sip of water as directed, has signed consent but says "I still have questions." Which cues require immediate action?

18. A patient receiving chemotherapy has: WBC 1,200/mm^3, temperature 99.8°F, no obvious source of infection on assessment, reports fatigue and mild nausea, has not had visitors in 2 days. Which finding is most concerning given the clinical context?

19. During a home health visit, you observe: patient's pillbox shows several missed doses this week, multiple expired medications in cabinet, patient seems confused about which medications to take when, lives alone, house is cluttered but not unsafe. Which cues indicate a medication management problem?

20. A patient reports new onset of "the worst headache of my life" that started suddenly 30 minutes ago. Other findings: BP 168/98, oriented but irritable, neck stiffness noted, photophobia present, no history of migraines. Which constellation of cues suggests a medical emergency?

CHAPTER 3

Analyze Cues

3.1 Overview

Analyzing cues is the second cognitive skill in the NCSBN Clinical Judgment Measurement Model (NCSBN, 2018). Once you have recognized relevant information, the next step is to determine what that information means. Analysis transforms raw data into clinical understanding—it is the bridge between observation and action.

If recognizing cues answers the question "What do I see?", analyzing cues answers "What does it mean?" This cognitive skill requires you to connect individual findings to each other, compare them to expected norms and the patient's baseline, and interpret their clinical significance. Effective analysis draws on your nursing knowledge, understanding of pathophysiology, and clinical experience.

Analysis is not a passive process of simply noting abnormalities. It requires active mental engagement—making connections, considering relationships, and constructing a coherent clinical picture from disparate pieces of information. This chapter will help you develop systematic approaches to cue analysis that will serve you throughout your nursing career.

3.2 The Purpose of Cue Analysis

Cue analysis serves several essential purposes in clinical judgment. Understanding these purposes will help you approach analysis more deliberately and effectively.

Making Sense of Complexity

Patients rarely present with single, isolated problems. More commonly, you will encounter multiple findings that may or may not be related to each other. A patient might have elevated blood pressure, anxiety, pain, and nausea simultaneously. Are these separate issues, or are they connected? Analysis helps you make sense of this complexity by identifying relationships among findings.

Consider a patient with the findings listed above. Through analysis, you might recognize that the elevated blood pressure and anxiety could both be responses to uncontrolled pain, and that the nausea might be a side effect of opioid medication given for that pain. Suddenly, what appeared to be four separate problems becomes one primary issue (pain) with secondary effects. This understanding fundamentally changes your approach to care.

Distinguishing Expected from Unexpected

Not every abnormal finding represents a problem requiring intervention. Some abnormalities are expected given the patient's condition or treatment. Analysis helps you distinguish between findings that are anticipated (even if technically abnormal) and those that signal a genuine clinical concern.

For example, a patient receiving chemotherapy is expected to have a decreased white blood cell count. This finding is abnormal compared to population norms but expected given the treatment. However, if that same patient develops a fever, the combination becomes significant—the expected immunosuppression plus the unexpected fever suggests possible infection in a vulnerable patient. Analysis considers context, not just absolute values.

Identifying Trends and Trajectories

A single data point tells you where a patient is at one moment; a series of data points reveals where they are heading. Analysis includes examining trends over time to determine whether a patient is improving, stable, or deteriorating. This trajectory information is often more clinically valuable than any single measurement.

A blood pressure of 100/60 mmHg might be acceptable in isolation, but if this patient's blood pressure has been steadily declining from 130/80 to 120/70 to 110/65 to 100/60 over the past few hours, the trend suggests a problem even though no single reading is dramatically abnormal. Effective analysis always considers the direction of change.

3.3 Clustering Related Data

One of the most important techniques in cue analysis is clustering—grouping related findings together to reveal patterns that might not be apparent when data is considered in isolation. Clustering helps you see the forest rather than just the trees.

What Is Clustering?

Clustering involves organizing assessment findings into meaningful groups based on their relationships. Findings can be clustered in several ways: by body system (all cardiovascular findings together), by potential problem (all findings that might indicate infection), by timeline (all changes that occurred in the last hour), or by relationship to a suspected condition.

The goal of clustering is pattern recognition. When you group related findings together, patterns emerge that point toward specific clinical problems. A single finding of tachycardia has many possible explanations, but when you cluster tachycardia with fever, elevated WBC, and localized redness and warmth, the pattern strongly suggests infection.

Clustering by Body System

Organizing findings by body system is a natural extension of systematic assessment. After completing your assessment, group all cardiovascular findings together, all respiratory findings together, and so on. This approach helps ensure you don't miss problems within a single system and makes it easier to identify system-specific issues.

Example: For a patient with potential cardiac problems, you might cluster: heart rate 110 and irregular, blood pressure 90/58, ECG showing atrial fibrillation, patient reports palpitations and dizziness, peripheral pulses weak. Grouped together, these findings clearly indicate a cardiovascular problem with hemodynamic compromise.

Clustering by Potential Problem

Another powerful approach is to cluster findings that might all relate to a suspected problem. This hypothesis-driven clustering helps you evaluate whether the evidence supports a particular clinical concern.

Example: If you suspect a patient might be developing sepsis, you would cluster: temperature 101.8°F (fever), heart rate 118 (tachycardia), respiratory rate 24 (tachypnea), blood pressure 88/56 (hypotension), WBC 18,000 (leukocytosis), lactate 3.2 (elevated), altered mental status. This cluster supports the sepsis hypothesis and indicates severity.

Clustering by Timeline

When a patient's condition changes, clustering findings by when they occurred can reveal cause-and-effect relationships or help identify a triggering event.

Example: A patient becomes acutely short of breath. You cluster recent events: received blood transfusion starting 30 minutes ago, developed itching 15 minutes ago, now has respiratory distress with wheezing, oxygen saturation dropping. The timeline clustering suggests transfusion reaction as the likely cause.

3.4 Identifying Patterns and Trends

Pattern recognition is at the heart of clinical expertise. Research on expert nurses shows that much of their clinical judgment relies on recognizing patterns they have encountered before (Benner, 1984). While this pattern library develops over years of practice, you can accelerate your learning by studying common clinical patterns and practicing pattern recognition deliberately.

Common Clinical Patterns

Certain clinical presentations occur frequently enough that they form recognizable patterns. Learning these patterns helps you quickly identify common problems. Here are several examples:

Fluid volume deficit pattern: Tachycardia, hypotension (especially orthostatic), decreased urine output, dry mucous membranes, poor skin turgor, elevated BUN/creatinine ratio, concentrated urine, thirst, weakness.

Fluid volume overload pattern: Weight gain, edema (peripheral or pulmonary), crackles in lungs, elevated JVP, S3 heart sound, dyspnea, orthopnea, decreased oxygen saturation.

Infection/sepsis pattern: Fever (or hypothermia in severe cases), tachycardia, tachypnea, elevated or very low WBC, altered mental status, hypotension, elevated lactate, source of infection (may or may not be apparent).

Respiratory distress pattern: Tachypnea, use of accessory muscles, nasal flaring, retractions, decreased oxygen saturation, abnormal breath sounds, inability to speak in full sentences, anxiety, tripod positioning.

Hypoglycemia pattern: Shakiness, diaphoresis, tachycardia, anxiety, confusion, irritability, hunger, pallor, weakness. In severe cases: seizures, loss of consciousness.

Opioid toxicity pattern: Decreased respiratory rate, decreased level of consciousness, pinpoint pupils (miosis), hypotension, bradycardia in severe cases.

Figure 3.1: Common Clinical Patterns Quick Reference

Common Clinical Patterns

Recognizing Cue Clusters That Suggest Specific Conditions

Pattern	Clustered Cues
Respiratory Distress	↑ RR, ↓ SpO2, accessory muscle use, nasal flaring, retractions, tripod positioning, inability to speak in full sentences, anxiety, cyanosis
Shock / Hypoperfusion	↓ BP, ↑ HR, weak/thready pulse, cool/clammy skin, pallor, delayed cap refill, ↓ urine output, altered LOC, restlessness, ↑ lactate
Infection / Sepsis	Fever OR hypothermia, ↑ HR, ↑ RR, ↑ WBC or ↓ WBC, chills, confusion (especially elderly), localized signs (redness, warmth, drainage), ↑ lactate, hypotension
Fluid Overload	Weight gain, edema (peripheral, sacral), JVD, crackles, dyspnea, orthopnea, S3 heart sound, ↑ BP, ↓ SpO2, bounding pulse, I>O
Dehydration / Hypovolemia	Dry mucous membranes, poor skin turgor, ↓ BP, ↑ HR, orthostatic hypotension, concentrated urine, ↓ urine output, thirst, weight loss, ↑ BUN/Cr ratio
Neurological Decline	↓ LOC, confusion, pupil changes, motor weakness, speech changes, ↓ GCS, headache, vomiting, seizures, Cushing's triad (↑BP, ↓HR, irregular RR)

Key Principle:
Individual cues may have multiple causes. When cues cluster together in recognizable patterns, they point toward specific conditions and guide your hypothesis generation.

When cues cluster together in recognizable patterns, they point toward specific conditions.

Analyzing Trends Over Time

Trends reveal trajectory—whether a patient is getting better, getting worse, or staying the same. To analyze trends effectively, you need multiple data points over time and must consider both the direction and rate of change.

Questions to guide trend analysis:

- How has this value changed from the patient's baseline?
- What is the direction of change (improving, worsening, stable)?
- How rapidly is the change occurring?
- Does the trend correlate with any intervention or event?
- If this trend continues, what would I expect to happen next?

Recognizing Deterioration

One of the most critical applications of trend analysis is recognizing patient deterioration early, before it becomes a crisis. Research shows that patients often display warning signs hours before cardiac arrest or other serious events, but these signs are frequently missed (Jones et al., 2013). Learning to recognize the pattern of deterioration can save lives.

Early warning signs of deterioration:

- Subtle changes in mental status (new confusion, agitation, lethargy)
- Increasing respiratory rate (often the earliest sign)
- Increasing heart rate
- Decreasing blood pressure
- Decreasing urine output
- Patient or family statement that something is "different" or "not right"
- Nurse intuition that something is wrong

3.5 Applying Nursing Knowledge to Analysis

Effective cue analysis requires you to connect assessment findings to your nursing knowledge base. This includes understanding normal physiology, pathophysiological processes, pharmacology, and the expected progression of common conditions. The more robust your knowledge base, the more effectively you can analyze clinical situations.

Using Pathophysiology

Understanding how diseases affect the body helps you predict what findings to expect and interpret what you observe. When you understand the pathophysiology of heart failure, for example, you understand why patients develop edema (fluid backs up due to decreased cardiac output), why they have crackles (fluid accumulates in lungs), and why they experience orthopnea (fluid redistributes when lying flat).

This pathophysiological understanding also helps you recognize when findings don't fit the expected pattern, which may indicate an additional problem or an alternative diagnosis. If a heart failure patient has the expected edema and crackles but also has a new fever and productive cough, the additional findings suggest a superimposed infection.

Considering Medications

Many clinical findings can be explained by medication effects—both intended therapeutic effects and unintended side effects or adverse reactions. Effective analysis always considers the patient's medication regimen.

A patient taking beta-blockers would be expected to have a lower heart rate, so a heart rate of 58 might be a therapeutic effect rather than a problem. A patient on diuretics might have low potassium. A patient recently started on ACE inhibitors might develop a dry cough. Including medication knowledge in your analysis helps you distinguish drug effects from disease processes.

Integrating Laboratory Data

Laboratory values provide objective data that can confirm or refute clinical suspicions. Effective analysis integrates lab results with physical assessment findings to build a complete picture.

When analyzing lab values, consider: Is this value normal or abnormal? How does it compare to previous values (trend)? Does it fit with the clinical picture suggested by other findings? Are there related lab values that should be checked? What is the clinical significance of this abnormality?

3.6 Clinical Application Examples

The following examples demonstrate cue analysis in clinical practice. Notice how clustering findings and applying nursing knowledge transforms raw data into clinical understanding.

Example 1: Postoperative Patient

Scenario: Mr. Adams, 67, is postoperative day 2 following colon resection. Assessment findings: T 101.4°F, HR 104, RR 22, BP 138/86. He reports increasing abdominal pain (now 7/10, was 4/10 yesterday). Abdomen is distended with hypoactive bowel sounds. He has not passed flatus since surgery. WBC is 14,500 (was 11,000 yesterday). Incision appears intact with minimal drainage.

Analysis: Clustering these findings reveals a concerning pattern. The fever plus rising WBC indicates an inflammatory or infectious process. The abdominal distension, absent flatus, and hypoactive bowel sounds suggest ileus or possible obstruction. The increasing pain is significant—postoperative pain typically improves by POD2, not worsens. Together, these findings raise concern for a possible surgical complication such as anastomotic leak, abscess, or developing peritonitis. This requires prompt physician notification.

Example 2: Cardiac Patient

Scenario: Mrs. Thompson, 78, admitted for heart failure exacerbation. Current findings: weight up 4 kg from admission weight 3 days ago despite diuretic therapy, 3+ pitting edema to knees (was 2+ to ankles), crackles now in lower half of lung fields bilaterally (were only at bases), SpO2 89% on 3L NC (was 94% on 2L yesterday), BNP 1,850 (was 1,200 on admission), patient reports worsening dyspnea.

Analysis: Every indicator is trending in the wrong direction despite treatment. The pattern clearly shows worsening fluid overload: increasing weight, worsening edema, worsening pulmonary congestion, declining oxygenation, rising BNP. The patient is not responding to current therapy. Analysis should prompt evaluation of diuretic effectiveness (is patient making urine?), consideration of medication adjustment, and assessment for factors that might be worsening heart failure (dietary indiscretion, medication non-compliance, new arrhythmia, ischemia).

Example 3: Medication Effect vs. Complication

Scenario: Mr. Chen, 55, started on a new blood pressure medication (lisinopril) one week ago. He reports a persistent dry cough that started a few days ago. Vital signs: BP 128/78 (previously 158/96), HR 72, RR 16. Lungs clear to auscultation. No fever, no sputum production, no shortness of breath. He feels well otherwise.

Analysis: The timing and characteristics of the cough suggest ACE inhibitor-induced cough, a known side effect of lisinopril occurring in 5-20% of patients. Supporting this interpretation: the cough is dry (not productive), there are no signs of respiratory infection (afebrile, lungs clear, no dyspnea), and it began shortly after starting the medication. The blood pressure response shows the medication is effective. This analysis would prompt discussion with the provider about whether to continue the medication, try a cough suppressant, or switch to an ARB.

3.7 Practice Problems (20)

For each scenario, analyze the cues provided. Cluster related findings, identify patterns, and explain what the data means clinically.

1. A patient has: HR 112, BP 88/54, RR 26, temperature 102.8°F, WBC 22,000, lactate 4.1, urine output 15 mL/hr for the past 3 hours, and appears confused (baseline is alert and oriented). Cluster these findings and identify the pattern.

2. A postpartum patient (day 2) has: fundus boggy and 2 cm above umbilicus, saturating one pad per hour with bright red blood, HR 118, BP 98/60 (baseline 120/74), patient reports feeling dizzy. What does this pattern suggest?

3. A diabetic patient has: blood glucose 52 mg/dL, skin cool and clammy, HR 108, confused and combative, last meal was 6 hours ago, took usual insulin dose. Analyze these findings.

4. An elderly patient has: new confusion (oriented x1), temperature 99.8°F, HR 92, urine cloudy with strong odor, WBC 13,800, patient recently completed antibiotics for bronchitis. What pattern do you recognize?

5. A patient with COPD has: SpO2 88% on room air, using accessory muscles, speaking in 2-3 word sentences, wheezing throughout lung fields, HR 108, has not used rescue inhaler today because "it ran out." Analyze these cues.

6. Post-cardiac catheterization patient has: right groin dressing with expanding area of blood (was 2 cm, now 6 cm in 1 hour), HR 110, BP 92/58, right leg cool compared to left, diminished right pedal pulse. What do these findings indicate?

7. A patient receiving a blood transfusion has: sudden onset of back pain, fever 102.4°F (was 98.6°F pre-transfusion), HR 118, BP 86/50, dark urine noted in Foley bag. Cluster and analyze.

8. A patient with cirrhosis has: increasing abdominal girth (up 3 cm from yesterday), new confusion, asterixis present, ammonia level 98, bilirubin 4.8, INR 2.1. What pattern is emerging?

9. A patient 4 hours post-thyroidectomy has: reports numbness and tingling around mouth and fingertips, positive Chvostek's sign, positive Trousseau's sign, calcium level pending. What complication does this suggest?

10. A trauma patient has: HR trending up (88→96→108→118 over 2 hours), BP trending down (130/82→118/76→108/68→96/62), decreasing urine output, skin pale and cool, patient increasingly anxious. Analyze the trend.

11. A patient with pneumonia (day 3 of antibiotics) has: temperature 98.8°F (was 101.6°F on admission), WBC 10,200 (was 16,400), SpO2 95% on room air (was 90% on 2L NC), cough less frequent, appetite improving. What does this trend indicate?

12. A patient on heparin infusion has: aPTT 98 seconds (therapeutic goal 60-80), bruising noted at IV sites, blood in urine, patient reports nosebleed this morning. Cluster and analyze.

13. A 3-day-old newborn has: weight down 12% from birth weight, 6 wet diapers in last 24 hours, jaundice visible to chest, bilirubin 16 mg/dL, mother reports difficulty with breastfeeding. Analyze these findings.

14. A patient with new onset atrial fibrillation has: HR 142 irregular, BP 104/68, reports palpitations and mild chest discomfort, slightly short of breath, no previous cardiac history. What does this pattern suggest about rate control?

15. A patient on day 5 of hospitalization has: temperature 100.8°F, new productive cough, right lower lobe crackles (lungs were clear on admission), WBC 14,200, SpO2 92% on RA. Patient has been mostly bed-bound. Analyze.

16. A patient with depression starting a new SSRI (day 10) has: increasing agitation, reports sleeping only 2 hours/night, pressured speech, reports "feeling better than ever," making impulsive financial decisions per family. Analyze this pattern.

17. A patient with recent hip replacement has: sudden onset chest pain and shortness of breath, HR 122, RR 28, SpO2 88% on RA, right calf tender and swollen (unilateral), patient appears anxious. What do these clustered findings suggest?

18. A patient taking digoxin has: HR 52, reports nausea and "seeing yellow halos around lights," potassium 3.1 mEq/L, digoxin level 2.8 ng/mL (therapeutic 0.8-2.0). Analyze these findings.

19. A patient with pancreatitis has: pain now 4/10 (was 9/10), tolerating clear liquids, bowel sounds present, amylase trending down (was 580, now 320), lipase trending down (was 890, now 410), afebrile. What does this trend indicate?

20. A patient admitted for alcohol detox (48 hours since last drink) has: visual hallucinations, tremors worsening despite benzodiazepines, HR 128, BP 168/102, temperature 100.6°F, diaphoretic. Analyze the severity of withdrawal.

CHAPTER 4

Prioritize Hypotheses

4.1 Overview

Prioritizing hypotheses is the third cognitive skill in the NCSBN Clinical Judgment Measurement Model (NCSBN, 2018). After recognizing relevant cues and analyzing their meaning, you must generate possible explanations for what is happening and determine which possibilities warrant the most urgent attention. This cognitive skill bridges assessment and action—it determines where you focus your clinical efforts.

A hypothesis in clinical practice is an educated explanation for a patient's signs, symptoms, or clinical presentation. Rarely does a set of findings point to only one possible cause. More commonly, several explanations are plausible, and you must determine which to consider first. Prioritization requires weighing both probability (what is most likely) and risk (what would be most dangerous if missed).

This chapter will help you develop systematic approaches to generating and prioritizing clinical hypotheses. Mastering this skill will help you avoid two common errors: tunnel vision (focusing too narrowly on one possibility) and analysis paralysis (being unable to move forward because too many possibilities seem equally valid).

4.2 Generating Hypotheses

Before you can prioritize, you must first generate a list of possible explanations for the patient's presentation. This requires both creative thinking (considering multiple possibilities) and disciplined reasoning (ensuring possibilities are clinically plausible given the available data).

Starting with the Data

Hypothesis generation should be driven by your assessment findings and analysis. Ask yourself: What conditions or problems could explain this cluster of findings? What diagnoses are consistent with this pattern? Consider the most common causes first, but also think about less common but serious possibilities that fit the clinical picture.

For example, if a patient presents with chest pain, shortness of breath, and diaphoresis, you would generate hypotheses that could explain all three findings: acute coronary syndrome, pulmonary embolism, aortic dissection, pneumothorax, or even severe anxiety. Each of these conditions can produce the observed symptoms, though with different likelihood and different implications.

Using Clinical Knowledge

Your nursing knowledge base is essential for generating appropriate hypotheses. Understanding pathophysiology helps you recognize which conditions produce which findings. Knowing risk factors helps you determine which conditions are more likely in a particular patient. Experience with common clinical presentations helps you recognize patterns quickly.

Consider the patient's context when generating hypotheses. A postoperative patient with fever suggests different possibilities than a patient with fever who just returned from international travel. A young, healthy patient with chest pain warrants different consideration than an elderly patient with multiple cardiac risk factors presenting with the same complaint.

Avoiding Premature Closure

One of the most dangerous cognitive errors in clinical reasoning is premature closure—settling on a diagnosis or explanation before adequately considering alternatives. This often happens when the first hypothesis that comes to mind seems to fit, and the clinician stops thinking about other possibilities.

To avoid premature closure, deliberately generate at least three possible explanations before deciding which is most likely. Ask yourself: What else could this be? What am I assuming? What would I be embarrassed to miss? This discipline helps ensure you don't overlook important possibilities, including rare but dangerous conditions.

4.3 The Probability vs. Risk Framework

Once you have generated possible hypotheses, you must prioritize them. The most effective framework for prioritization considers two dimensions: probability (how likely is this explanation?) and risk (how dangerous would it be to miss this diagnosis?).

Figure 4.1: Probability vs. Risk Prioritization Matrix

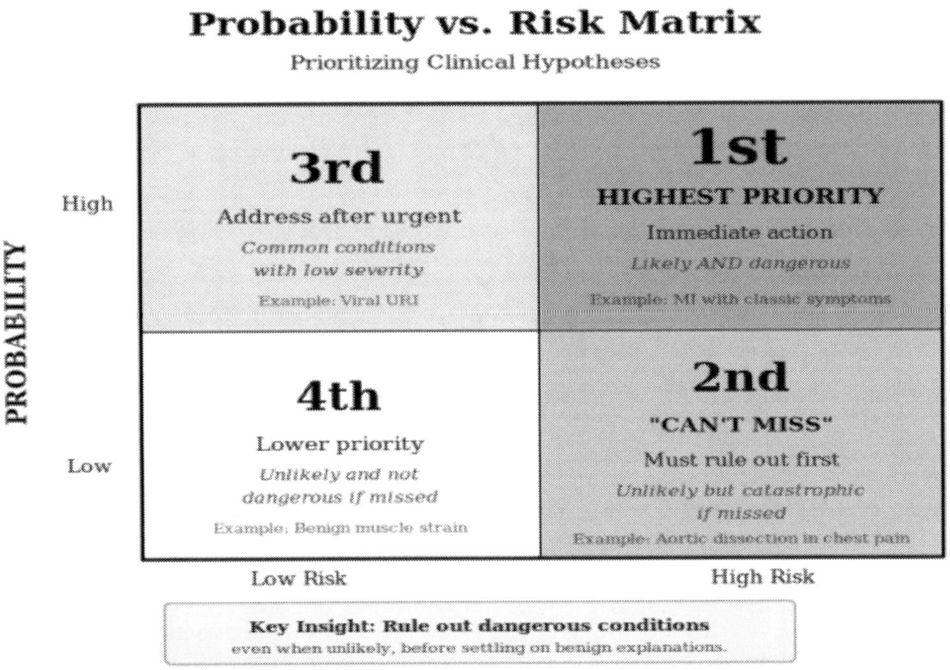

High-risk conditions may warrant priority attention even when probability is relatively low.

Assessing Probability

Probability assessment asks: Given the available evidence, how likely is each hypothesis to be correct? Several factors influence probability:

Prevalence. Common conditions are more likely than rare ones. In medicine, there is a saying: "When you hear hoofbeats, think horses, not zebras." Most patients with headache have tension headache or migraine, not brain tumors. This doesn't mean you ignore rare possibilities, but common diagnoses deserve primary consideration.

Fit with findings. How well does each hypothesis explain all the observed findings? A hypothesis that accounts for most or all findings is more likely than one that explains only some. If findings don't fit the suspected diagnosis, consider whether an additional problem exists or whether the primary hypothesis is wrong.

Risk factors. A patient's risk factors shift probability. A lifelong smoker with weight loss and hemoptysis has a higher probability of lung cancer than a young nonsmoker with the same symptoms. Consider the patient's age, comorbidities, medications, lifestyle, and history.

Clinical course. How the patient's condition has evolved provides important probability information. Sudden onset suggests different diagnoses than gradual progression. Improvement with treatment supports the working diagnosis; failure to improve suggests reconsideration.

Assessing Risk

Risk assessment asks: What are the consequences if this hypothesis is correct and I miss it or delay treatment? Some conditions are dangerous primarily because of what happens if they are not treated promptly. Others are dangerous because of their natural progression regardless of treatment.

Time-sensitivity. Some conditions deteriorate rapidly without treatment. Acute myocardial infarction, stroke, sepsis, and anaphylaxis are examples where delays of even minutes can significantly affect outcomes. These time-sensitive conditions warrant high priority even when probability is moderate.

Severity of outcome. Consider what happens if the diagnosis is missed. Will the patient die? Suffer permanent disability? Experience significant morbidity? A missed diagnosis of tension headache has very different consequences than a missed diagnosis of subarachnoid hemorrhage.

Treatability. Conditions that are treatable if caught early but devastating if missed deserve high priority. A pulmonary embolism is life-threatening if untreated but highly treatable with anticoagulation. This treatability increases the importance of not missing the diagnosis.

Balancing Probability and Risk

The key insight of the probability-risk framework is that high-risk conditions may warrant priority attention even when their probability is relatively low. Consider the following principle: Always rule out the "can't miss" diagnoses before settling on a more benign explanation.

For example, a young patient with chest pain most likely has a musculoskeletal problem or anxiety. However, acute coronary syndrome, pulmonary embolism, and aortic dissection—though less common in young patients—are life-threatening if missed. The prudent approach is to evaluate for these dangerous possibilities before attributing the pain to a benign cause.

4.4 Prioritization Frameworks

Several established frameworks can guide your prioritization thinking. These frameworks provide structure for ensuring you address the most critical concerns first.

ABCs: Airway, Breathing, Circulation

The ABCs represent the most fundamental prioritization framework in healthcare. Any threat to airway, breathing, or circulation takes precedence over other concerns because these are immediately life-threatening. When multiple hypotheses exist, those involving ABC compromise are addressed first.

This framework reminds us that physiological stability is the prerequisite for addressing other problems. A patient cannot benefit from treatment of their underlying condition if they cannot maintain adequate oxygenation and perfusion. Stabilize first, then diagnose and treat.

Maslow's Hierarchy of Needs

Maslow's hierarchy, adapted for nursing, provides a broader prioritization framework. Physiological needs (oxygen, circulation, nutrition, elimination, temperature regulation) take precedence over safety needs, which take precedence over love/belonging, which take precedence over esteem, which take precedence over self-actualization.

In clinical application, this means addressing physical survival needs before psychological needs, and basic safety before higher-level concerns. A patient in respiratory distress needs oxygen before education about their condition. A patient in pain needs relief before discussing discharge planning.

Figure 4.2: Maslow's Hierarchy in Nursing Prioritization

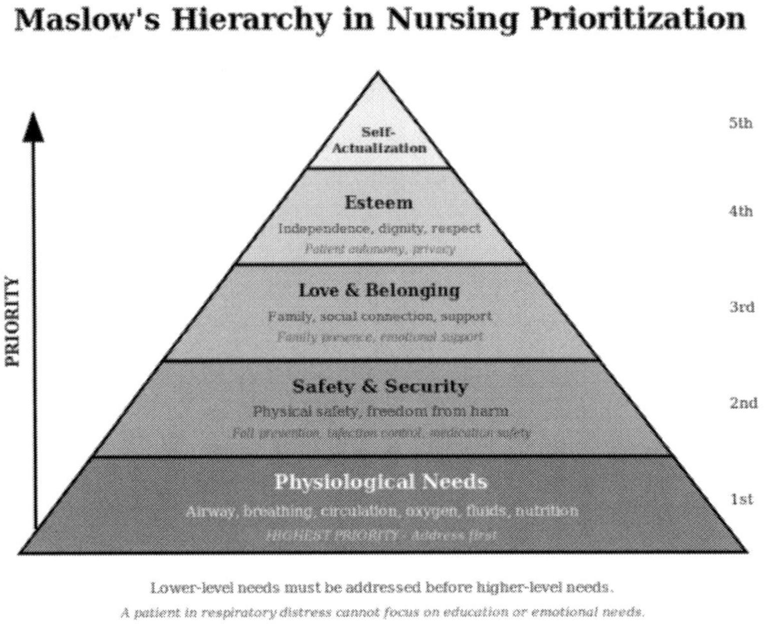

Lower-level needs must be addressed before higher-level needs.

Acute vs. Chronic

Acute problems generally take priority over chronic ones. A new symptom or sudden change warrants more immediate attention than a longstanding, stable condition. This is because acute changes may signal deterioration requiring urgent intervention, while chronic problems have already demonstrated relative stability.

However, this framework has nuances. An acute exacerbation of a chronic condition may be more serious than a new but minor acute problem. Context matters. The key question is: What requires attention right now to prevent harm?

Actual vs. Potential Problems

Actual problems—those currently present—generally take priority over potential problems—those that might develop. A patient who is actively bleeding needs intervention before a patient who is at risk for bleeding. However, high-risk potential problems may warrant preventive action, especially when the potential consequence is severe and prevention is feasible.

4.5 Clinical Application of Prioritization

Applying prioritization in clinical practice requires integrating all these considerations—probability, risk, frameworks—while remaining flexible as new information emerges. The following examples illustrate this process.

Example 1: Chest Pain in the Emergency Department

Scenario: A 58-year-old man presents with substernal chest pressure radiating to his left arm, diaphoresis, and nausea. He has a history of hypertension and hyperlipidemia. Vital signs: HR 96, BP 158/94, RR 20, SpO2 97%.

Possible hypotheses: (1) Acute coronary syndrome/MI, (2) Unstable angina, (3) Aortic dissection, (4) Pulmonary embolism, (5) GERD/esophageal spasm, (6) Musculoskeletal pain, (7) Anxiety/panic attack.

Prioritization rationale: ACS/MI is the highest priority—the presentation is classic, risk factors are present, and missing this diagnosis can be fatal. Aortic dissection is second priority as it can mimic MI but requires different treatment (anticoagulation for MI would be catastrophic in dissection). PE is third. These "must not miss" diagnoses are evaluated before considering GERD, musculoskeletal, or anxiety causes, even though these benign causes are statistically more common in the general population.

Example 2: Postoperative Fever

Scenario: A patient is postoperative day 3 following abdominal surgery. She develops a fever of 101.8°F with mild tachycardia. She reports some incisional tenderness and has a Foley catheter and peripheral IV in place.

Possible hypotheses: Using the "5 W's" of postoperative fever: (1) Wind—atelectasis/pneumonia, (2) Water—UTI, (3) Wound—surgical site infection, (4) Walking—DVT/PE, (5) Wonder drugs—medication reaction or C. difficile.

Prioritization rationale: On POD3, the timing shifts probability. Atelectasis typically causes fever in the first 48 hours, so it's less likely now. UTI and wound infection become more probable by day 3-5. DVT/PE must always be considered in postoperative patients, especially if immobile. Priorities: (1) Assess for PE if any respiratory symptoms (high risk), (2) Examine wound for signs of SSI, (3) Assess urine for UTI signs, (4) Lung assessment for pneumonia, (5) Review medications and stool frequency.

Example 3: Altered Mental Status

Scenario: An 82-year-old nursing home resident is brought to the hospital for "acting confused" for the past day. She is normally alert and oriented. Current findings: temperature 99.4°F, HR 92, BP 108/62, glucose 118, appears drowsy and disoriented.

Possible hypotheses: Using a delirium workup approach: (1) Infection (UTI, pneumonia, skin), (2) Medications (new drug, dosage change, polypharmacy), (3) Metabolic (electrolytes, renal/hepatic function, thyroid), (4) Hypoxia, (5) Cardiac (MI can present atypically in elderly), (6) Neurological (stroke, subdural hematoma), (7) Urinary retention, (8) Constipation/impaction.

Prioritization rationale: In elderly patients with acute confusion, infection is the most common cause—UTI leads the list. However, stroke and MI present atypically in the elderly and are "can't miss" diagnoses. Priorities: (1) Rule out stroke (time-sensitive), (2) ECG to evaluate for MI, (3) Urinalysis for UTI (most common), (4) Comprehensive metabolic panel, (5) Medication reconciliation, (6) Bladder scan for retention, (7) Chest X-ray if any respiratory findings.

4.6 Practice Problems (20)

For each scenario, generate at least three possible hypotheses and prioritize them, explaining your rationale based on probability and risk.

1. A 45-year-old woman presents with sudden onset of severe headache, describing it as "the worst headache of my life." She has nausea and mild neck stiffness. Vital signs are stable except BP 162/98. Generate and prioritize hypotheses.

2. A 6-month-old infant is brought in by parents for "not acting right." The baby is irritable, has a temperature of 102.4°F, and has had decreased feeding. The fontanelle appears slightly bulging. Generate and prioritize hypotheses.

3. A 70-year-old man with COPD presents with worsening shortness of breath over 3 days. He has increased sputum production (now yellow-green), mild fever, and SpO2 88% on room air. He also reports bilateral leg swelling. Generate and prioritize hypotheses.

4. A 28-year-old woman presents with sharp chest pain that worsens with deep breathing. She started oral contraceptives 2 months ago and recently took a 6-hour car trip. HR 108, RR 22, SpO2 94%. Generate and prioritize hypotheses.

5. A 55-year-old diabetic man presents with left foot redness, warmth, and swelling. He has a small ulcer on the sole of his foot. Temperature 101.2°F, glucose 286, WBC 16,400. Generate and prioritize hypotheses.

6. A postoperative patient (day 1 after hip replacement) becomes acutely short of breath with chest pain. HR 118, BP 92/58, SpO2 86% on room air. The right leg is more swollen than the left. Generate and prioritize hypotheses.

7. A 35-year-old woman presents with fatigue, weight gain, constipation, and feeling cold all the time. Her skin appears dry and she has mild periorbital edema. HR 56, BP 98/64. Generate and prioritize hypotheses.

8. A 78-year-old man is found on the floor by his daughter. He is confused, has slurred speech, and cannot move his right arm or leg. His daughter saw him "normal" 2 hours ago. BP 188/102. Generate and prioritize hypotheses.

9. A 22-year-old college student presents with fever, severe sore throat, fatigue, and swollen lymph nodes in her neck. She has a grayish coating on her tonsils. HR 98, temperature 102.8°F. Generate and prioritize hypotheses.

10. A 65-year-old woman presents with sudden onset of abdominal pain, nausea, and vomiting. She has a history of atrial fibrillation and is not compliant with anticoagulation. Abdomen is diffusely tender with guarding. Generate and prioritize hypotheses.

11. A 40-year-old man presents with severe epigastric pain radiating to his back, nausea, and vomiting. He admits to heavy alcohol use over the past week. Temperature 100.4°F, HR 110, BP 138/88. Generate and prioritize hypotheses.

12. A 3-year-old child presents with barking cough, stridor at rest, and mild respiratory distress. Symptoms started suddenly tonight. No fever. No history of choking episode. Generate and prioritize hypotheses.

13. A 50-year-old woman on chemotherapy presents with temperature 100.8°F, WBC 800/mm^3, and no obvious source of infection. She feels fatigued but has no focal symptoms. Generate and prioritize hypotheses.

14. A 25-year-old man presents with progressive weakness over 2 weeks, starting in his legs and now affecting his arms. He had a "stomach bug" 3 weeks ago. Deep tendon reflexes are diminished. Generate and prioritize hypotheses.

15. A 68-year-old woman presents with painless jaundice, dark urine, and clay-colored stools. She has lost 15 pounds over 2 months without trying. No abdominal pain. Generate and prioritize hypotheses.

16. A 30-year-old pregnant woman (32 weeks) presents with headache, visual changes, and right upper quadrant pain. BP 168/110, protein in urine. She has gained 5 pounds this week. Generate and prioritize hypotheses.

17. A 60-year-old man with known heart failure presents with worsening shortness of breath, weight gain, and inability to lie flat. He also mentions pink, frothy sputum this morning. HR 112, RR 28, SpO2 84% on room air. Generate and prioritize hypotheses.

18. An 18-year-old woman presents with lower abdominal pain, vaginal discharge, and pain with urination. She is sexually active with a new partner. Temperature 101°F, lower abdominal tenderness with palpation. Generate and prioritize hypotheses.

19. A 72-year-old man presents with syncope. He reports feeling his "heart racing" before passing out. He regained consciousness within seconds. ECG shows atrial fibrillation with rate of 150. Generate and prioritize hypotheses.

20. A 45-year-old man presents with progressive difficulty swallowing over 6 months, now having trouble with liquids as well as solids. He has lost 20 pounds. No pain with swallowing. He has a history of long-standing GERD. Generate and prioritize hypotheses.

CHAPTER 5

Generate Solutions

5.1 Overview

Generating solutions is the fourth cognitive skill in the NCSBN Clinical Judgment Measurement Model (NCSBN, 2018). After recognizing cues, analyzing their meaning, and prioritizing hypotheses about what is happening, you must identify potential interventions to address the patient's needs. This cognitive skill transforms your clinical understanding into a plan for action.

Generating solutions is not simply selecting the first intervention that comes to mind. It requires you to consider multiple options, weigh their potential benefits and risks, and select interventions that are appropriate for this specific patient in this specific situation. The best solution for one patient may not be the best solution for another patient with the same problem.

This chapter will help you develop a systematic approach to identifying appropriate nursing interventions. You will learn to draw on evidence-based practice, consider available resources, anticipate potential complications, and select interventions that address both the immediate problem and the patient's broader needs.

5.2 Types of Nursing Interventions

Nursing interventions can be categorized in several ways. Understanding these categories helps ensure you consider the full range of options available to address patient needs.

Independent Nursing Interventions

Independent interventions are those that nurses can initiate based on their own clinical judgment without a physician order. These interventions fall within the scope of nursing practice and are based on nursing knowledge and assessment. Examples include:

- Repositioning a patient to prevent pressure injuries
- Elevating the head of bed to improve breathing
- Implementing fall precautions based on risk assessment
- Providing patient education about disease management
- Applying ice or heat for comfort
- Assisting with ambulation to prevent complications
- Providing emotional support and therapeutic communication

Independent interventions represent a significant portion of nursing care and demonstrate the autonomous nature of nursing practice. Skilled nurses recognize opportunities to implement independent interventions that prevent complications and promote recovery.

Dependent Nursing Interventions

Dependent interventions require a physician or other authorized prescriber's order before implementation. While nurses cannot independently initiate these interventions, nurses play crucial roles in identifying the need for them, communicating with prescribers, implementing orders safely, and monitoring patient response. Examples include:

- Administering prescribed medications
- Implementing ordered IV fluid therapy
- Carrying out prescribed treatments (wound care per protocol, etc.)
- Applying ordered medical devices (oxygen, catheters, etc.)
- Performing ordered diagnostic tests

When generating solutions, nurses often identify the need for dependent interventions and must communicate effectively with prescribers to obtain appropriate orders. This communication is itself a nursing skill—knowing what to ask for, how to present information persuasively, and when to escalate concerns.

Collaborative Interventions

Collaborative interventions involve working with other healthcare team members to address patient needs. Modern healthcare is inherently team-based, and many patient problems require coordinated efforts across disciplines. Examples include:

- Consulting respiratory therapy for breathing treatments
- Coordinating with physical therapy for mobility goals
- Working with dietary services for nutritional interventions
- Engaging social work for discharge planning needs
- Consulting wound care specialists for complex wounds
- Involving case management for care coordination

Effective nurses know when to involve other team members and how to coordinate care across disciplines. Recognizing the limits of your own expertise and engaging appropriate resources is a sign of professional maturity, not weakness.

5.3 Evidence-Based Practice

Evidence-based practice (EBP) is the conscientious integration of best available research evidence with clinical expertise and patient values to make decisions about patient care (Melnyk & Fineout-Overholt, 2019). When generating solutions, your interventions should be grounded in evidence whenever possible.

Why Evidence Matters

Healthcare has a long history of interventions that seemed logical but were later proven ineffective or harmful. Evidence-based practice protects patients by ensuring that interventions have been tested and shown to work. It also protects nurses by providing a rationale for clinical decisions that can be articulated and defended.

Evidence exists on a hierarchy, from strongest to weakest: systematic reviews and meta-analyses at the top, followed by randomized controlled trials, cohort studies, case-control studies, case series, and expert opinion at the bottom. While high-quality evidence isn't available for every clinical question, nurses should seek the best available evidence to guide their practice.

Applying Evidence to Individual Patients

Evidence from research provides general guidance, but each patient is unique. Applying evidence requires considering how the individual patient's circumstances, preferences, and values affect which interventions are appropriate. A treatment that is effective on average may not be the right choice for a specific patient due to contraindications, patient preferences, or practical constraints.

For example, research may show that a particular medication is the most effective treatment for a condition, but if your patient cannot afford it, has a contraindication, or strongly prefers an alternative approach, the "best" evidence-based option may not be the best choice for that patient. Clinical judgment involves integrating evidence with patient-specific factors.

Clinical Practice Guidelines

Clinical practice guidelines translate research evidence into specific recommendations for practice. These guidelines, developed by professional organizations and expert panels, can be valuable resources when generating solutions. Examples include guidelines from the American Heart Association for cardiac care, the Surviving Sepsis Campaign for sepsis management, and the Wound, Ostomy and Continence Nurses Society for wound care.

Familiarity with guidelines relevant to your practice area strengthens your ability to generate evidence-based solutions. However, guidelines should inform clinical judgment, not replace it. Guidelines are developed for typical patients; your patient may have unique circumstances that warrant deviation from standard recommendations.

5.4 Considering Resources and Constraints

Ideal solutions are not always feasible solutions. When generating interventions, you must consider the resources available and the constraints that may limit your options. Practical clinical judgment means identifying solutions that are not only clinically appropriate but also implementable in your specific context.

Available Resources

Resources that affect solution generation include:

Equipment and supplies. What monitoring equipment, medical devices, and supplies are available? A solution requiring equipment that isn't available is not practical. Knowing what resources exist on your unit helps you generate feasible interventions.

Medications. What medications are available, either from unit stock or through pharmacy? In emergencies, some medications may not be immediately accessible. Knowing what is available for urgent use affects intervention selection.

Personnel. What staff members are available to assist? Some interventions require multiple people. Others require specialized expertise. Consider who is available and what skills they bring.

Time. How much time is available? Emergency situations demand rapid interventions. Non-urgent situations allow more deliberate planning. The acuity of the situation affects which solutions are appropriate.

Patient-Specific Factors

Patient factors that influence solution selection include:

Allergies and contraindications. What interventions are ruled out by patient allergies or medical contraindications? Always check before selecting medication interventions.

Comorbidities. How do the patient's other medical conditions affect intervention selection? An intervention safe for most patients may be risky for patients with certain comorbidities.

Patient preferences. What does the patient want? Patient autonomy means respecting patient choices, even when they differ from what you might recommend. Understand patient goals and values.

Functional status. What is the patient capable of doing? Interventions requiring patient participation must match patient abilities. Consider mobility, cognition, and self-care capacity.

Social support. What support does the patient have? Discharge planning interventions must consider who will assist the patient at home. Complex home treatments require capable caregivers.

Anticipating Complications

When generating solutions, think ahead to potential complications and have contingency plans ready. What could go wrong with your planned intervention? What will you do if it doesn't work? What side effects or adverse reactions should you monitor for?

Experienced nurses plan not only their primary intervention but also their backup plan. If the first-line treatment fails, what is the next option? This anticipatory thinking helps you respond quickly when situations don't go as planned.

5.5 The Solution Generation Process

Generating solutions is a systematic process that can be approached through a series of questions. Working through these questions helps ensure you consider the full range of options and select the most appropriate interventions.

Step 1: What is the priority problem? Based on your hypothesis prioritization, identify the most urgent issue to address. Your solutions should target this priority first.

Step 2: What does the evidence suggest? What interventions have been shown to be effective for this problem? Consider guidelines, research, and established best practices.

Step 3: What independent interventions can I implement now? What actions can you take immediately without waiting for orders? These nursing interventions can often be started while awaiting physician response.

Step 4: What orders do I need to request? What dependent interventions are indicated? Prepare to communicate clearly with prescribers about what you need and why.

Step 5: Who else needs to be involved? What other team members should be engaged? Consider consultations, referrals, and collaborative interventions.

Step 6: What are the patient's preferences? How do the patient's values and wishes affect the plan? Ensure patient involvement in decision-making when possible.

Step 7: What is my backup plan? If the primary intervention fails or is unavailable, what is the alternative? Anticipate contingencies.

5.6 Clinical Application Examples

The following examples demonstrate solution generation in clinical practice. Notice how the nurse considers multiple intervention types, weighs options, and selects approaches tailored to the specific situation.

Example 1: Hypoglycemia

Scenario: A diabetic patient has a blood glucose of 58 mg/dL and is symptomatic with shakiness and diaphoresis but is alert and able to swallow.

Solution generation:

Priority problem: Hypoglycemia requiring immediate glucose replacement.

Independent interventions: Administer 15-20g fast-acting carbohydrate (juice, glucose tablets) per facility protocol—the "Rule of 15." Stay with patient, recheck glucose in 15 minutes.

Dependent interventions: If patient cannot take oral intake or does not respond, IV dextrose or glucagon will be needed—check for orders, prepare to request if not available.

Collaborative: May need dietary consult if recurrent hypoglycemia suggests meal planning issues. May need pharmacy consult for insulin regimen adjustment.

Patient factors: Patient is alert and can swallow, so oral route is appropriate. Check for contraindications to sugary drinks.

Backup plan: If patient becomes unresponsive, switch to IV D50 or glucagon. Have emergency equipment accessible.

Example 2: Respiratory Distress

Scenario: A patient with COPD develops increased shortness of breath with SpO2 of 86% on room air, respiratory rate of 28, and use of accessory muscles.

Solution generation:

Priority problem: Hypoxemia and increased work of breathing.

Independent interventions: Position patient upright (high Fowler's or tripod position), remain calm to reduce patient anxiety, prepare for escalation. Encourage pursed-lip breathing.

Dependent interventions: Apply supplemental oxygen per protocol (titrate carefully in COPD—target SpO2 88-92%), request PRN bronchodilator if available, notify provider for orders.

Collaborative: Respiratory therapy for nebulizer treatments and possible BiPAP. Physician for evaluation and possible steroids.

Patient factors: COPD history means hypoxic drive may be present—avoid over-oxygenation. Check for recent medication compliance, infections, triggers.

Backup plan: If patient continues deteriorating despite interventions, prepare for possible intubation. Know location of crash cart and rapid response activation.

Example 3: Post-Surgical Pain

Scenario: A postoperative patient reports pain of 8/10 despite receiving scheduled acetaminophen. The patient has a PRN order for hydrocodone but is concerned about taking opioids because her mother was addicted.

Solution generation:

Priority problem: Uncontrolled acute pain affecting recovery.

Independent interventions: Provide reassurance about appropriate short-term opioid use vs. addiction, reposition for comfort, apply ice if appropriate, offer distraction techniques, assess pain characteristics.

Dependent interventions: Discuss patient concerns with her before administering opioid, request alternative non-opioid options from provider if patient refuses opioids (ketorolac, gabapentin, etc.).

Collaborative: May need pain management consult if multimodal approach needed. Consider integrative approaches if available.

Patient factors: Patient's family history and concerns must be respected. Education about difference between dependence, tolerance, and addiction. Shared decision-making is essential.

Backup plan: If patient declines all pharmacological options, maximize non-pharmacological approaches and document informed refusal.

5.7 Practice Problems (20)

For each scenario, generate appropriate solutions. Consider independent, dependent, and collaborative interventions. Identify the priority intervention and explain your rationale.

1. A patient with heart failure has gained 4 pounds overnight and has increased bilateral lower extremity edema. SpO2 is 92% on room air, and the patient reports mild dyspnea. What solutions should you generate?

2. An elderly patient is becoming increasingly confused and agitated. You suspect delirium. The patient has pulled out their IV twice and is attempting to climb out of bed. What interventions should you consider?

3. A patient with diabetes has a foot ulcer that is not healing despite 2 weeks of treatment. The wound has increased drainage and mild surrounding redness. Blood glucose has been poorly controlled. What solutions should you generate?

4. A postoperative patient has not voided in 10 hours despite adequate fluid intake. They report lower abdominal pressure but cannot urinate. Bladder scan shows 650 mL. What interventions should you consider?

5. A patient receiving IV antibiotics develops a rash and reports itching. Vital signs are stable, and there is no respiratory distress or swelling. What solutions should you generate?

6. A patient admitted for pneumonia has thick secretions and a weak, ineffective cough. SpO2 is 91% on 2L nasal cannula. Lung sounds reveal crackles and rhonchi throughout. What interventions should you consider?

7. A patient with a history of falls is insisting on getting up to the bathroom independently. They have an unsteady gait and have fallen twice at home in the past month. What solutions should you generate?

8. A newly diagnosed cancer patient is tearful and says "I just found out and I don't know what to do. I can't even think straight." What interventions should you consider?

9. A patient on anticoagulation for atrial fibrillation has an INR of 5.2 (therapeutic goal 2-3). There are no signs of active bleeding. What solutions should you generate?

10. A breastfeeding mother is reporting severe nipple pain and has visible cracks with slight bleeding. Her baby is one week old. What interventions should you consider?

11. A patient with chronic kidney disease has a potassium level of 6.2 mEq/L. They have no ECG changes but report mild muscle weakness. What solutions should you generate?

12. A patient preparing for discharge after a myocardial infarction expresses concern about resuming sexual activity. They are embarrassed to ask their doctor. What interventions should you consider?

13. A patient with a nasogastric tube for bowel obstruction is having significant nausea despite the NG tube. The tube is draining green fluid, but the patient feels no relief. What solutions should you generate?

14. An 85-year-old patient who was independent at home is being discharged after hip replacement. They live alone and have 10 stairs to enter their home. What interventions should you consider?

15. A patient with bipolar disorder who has been stable on lithium is showing signs of toxicity: tremor, nausea, diarrhea, and confusion. Lithium level is pending. What solutions should you generate?

16. A patient with severe COPD is being discharged on home oxygen for the first time. They live with a family member who smokes. What interventions should you consider?

17. A patient with cirrhosis has increasing abdominal girth and is becoming short of breath due to ascites. They have had 2 liters removed via paracentesis 5 days ago. What solutions should you generate?

18. A pediatric patient, age 4, needs an IV started for antibiotic therapy. The child is extremely anxious, crying, and clinging to their parent. What interventions should you consider?

19. A patient with Parkinson's disease is having difficulty swallowing their medications. Several pills were found partially dissolved on their tongue after they thought they had swallowed them. What solutions should you generate?

20. A patient with a Stage 3 pressure injury to the sacrum requires dressing changes that cause significant pain despite premedication. The current treatment plan requires daily dressing changes. What interventions should you consider?

CHAPTER 6

Take Action

6.1 Overview

Taking action is the fifth cognitive skill in the NCSBN Clinical Judgment Measurement Model (NCSBN, 2018). After recognizing cues, analyzing their meaning, prioritizing hypotheses, and generating solutions, you must implement your chosen interventions effectively. This is where clinical judgment translates into clinical care—where thinking becomes doing.

Taking action encompasses more than simply performing a task. It involves prioritizing when multiple actions are needed, delegating appropriately to other team members, communicating effectively with patients and colleagues, ensuring safety throughout the process, and documenting your actions accurately. Each of these components is essential to effective implementation.

This chapter will help you develop skills in implementing nursing interventions safely and effectively. You will learn frameworks for prioritizing actions, principles of delegation, strategies for clear communication, and best practices for documentation. These skills ensure that your well-reasoned clinical judgments result in high-quality patient care.

6.2 Prioritizing Actions

When a patient has multiple needs or when you are caring for multiple patients, you must determine which actions to take first. Prioritization ensures that the most critical needs are addressed before less urgent ones. Several frameworks guide this prioritization.

The ABCs: Airway, Breathing, Circulation

The ABC framework is the most fundamental prioritization tool in healthcare. When assessing what to do first, always consider: Is the airway patent? Is breathing adequate? Is circulation sufficient? Problems in these areas are immediately life-threatening and take precedence over all other concerns.

In some situations, this framework expands to ABCDE: Airway, Breathing, Circulation, Disability (neurological status), and Exposure (full assessment/temperature control). The principle remains the same—address immediate threats to survival first, in order of their impact on life.

Figure 6.1: ABCs and ABCDE Prioritization

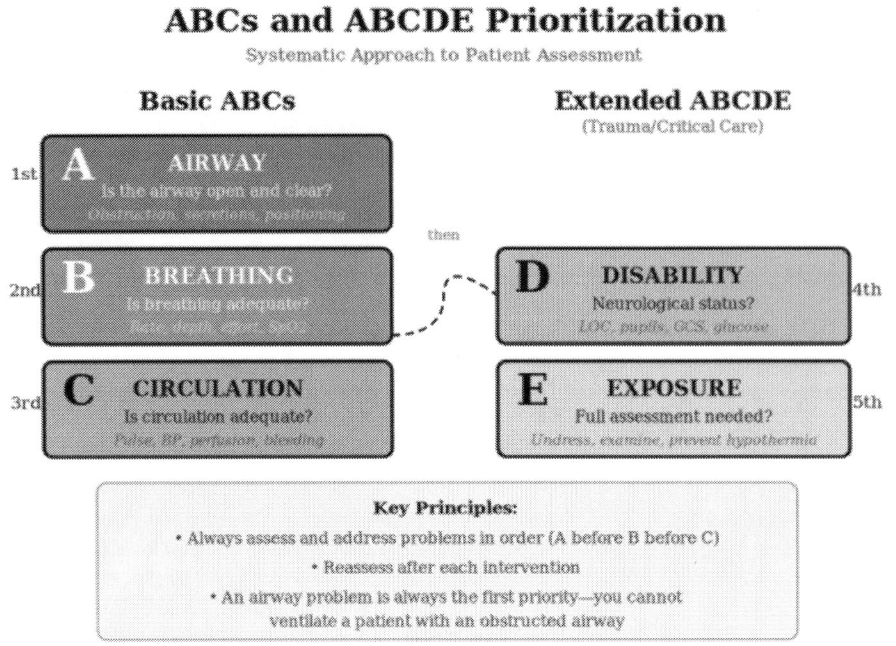

Always assess and address problems in ABC order—an airway problem is always the first priority.

Maslow's Hierarchy Applied to Nursing

Maslow's hierarchy of needs provides a broader framework for prioritization. In nursing application, the hierarchy suggests addressing needs in this order:

1. Physiological needs (oxygen, fluids, nutrition, elimination, rest, comfort)
2. Safety and security needs (physical safety, psychological security)
3. Love and belonging needs (relationships, family involvement)
4. Esteem needs (dignity, independence, achievement)
5. Self-actualization needs (growth, reaching potential)

This framework helps when the ABCs are stable but multiple needs compete for attention. Address basic physiological and safety needs before higher-level concerns. A patient cannot focus on education about their condition (higher-level need) if they are in pain (physiological need) or afraid (safety need).

Acute Before Chronic

New, acute problems generally take priority over chronic, stable conditions. A sudden change in patient status demands immediate attention, while a longstanding issue that has been stable can often wait. The exception is when a chronic condition is decompensating—then it becomes an acute priority.

Unstable Before Stable

Patients whose conditions are unstable or changing require more immediate attention than stable patients. When prioritizing among multiple patients, assess who is most unstable and address their needs first. Stable patients can often wait briefly while you attend to urgent situations.

Prioritization in Practice

In real clinical situations, prioritization often requires balancing multiple frameworks. Consider this example: You have four patients. Patient A needs pain medication (pain 6/10, chronic condition). Patient B's IV pump is beeping (bag empty). Patient C's family has questions about discharge. Patient D just rang the call bell reporting sudden shortness of breath.

Using prioritization principles: Patient D takes priority—sudden respiratory change is an acute, potentially life-threatening situation (ABCs). Patient B is next—while an empty IV bag isn't immediately dangerous, the patient may be receiving critical medications. Patient A is next—pain is a physiological need but is chronic and rated moderate. Patient C is last—discharge questions are important but not urgent.

6.3 Delegation

Delegation is the transfer of responsibility for performing a task to another person while retaining accountability for the outcome. Effective delegation is essential for managing patient care efficiently, but it requires careful judgment about what can be delegated, to whom, and under what circumstances.

The Five Rights of Delegation

The National Council of State Boards of Nursing identifies five rights of delegation that guide appropriate delegation decisions (NCSBN, 2016):

Right task. Is this task appropriate to delegate? Some tasks must be performed by licensed nurses and cannot be delegated. Tasks that are routine, require minimal judgment, and have predictable outcomes are more appropriate for delegation.

Right circumstance. Is delegation appropriate given the patient's current condition and the care setting? A task that could be delegated for a stable patient may not be appropriate for an unstable patient.

Right person. Is the delegatee qualified and competent to perform this task? Consider training, experience, and demonstrated competency. The right person must also be the right level—some tasks can go to UAPs, others only to LPNs/LVNs.

Right direction/communication. Have you provided clear, specific instructions? The delegatee must understand what to do, how to do it, when to report back, and what findings require immediate notification.

Right supervision. Are you providing appropriate oversight? Delegation does not mean abandonment. You remain accountable for the outcome and must monitor that the task is completed appropriately.

Figure 6.2: Five Rights of Delegation

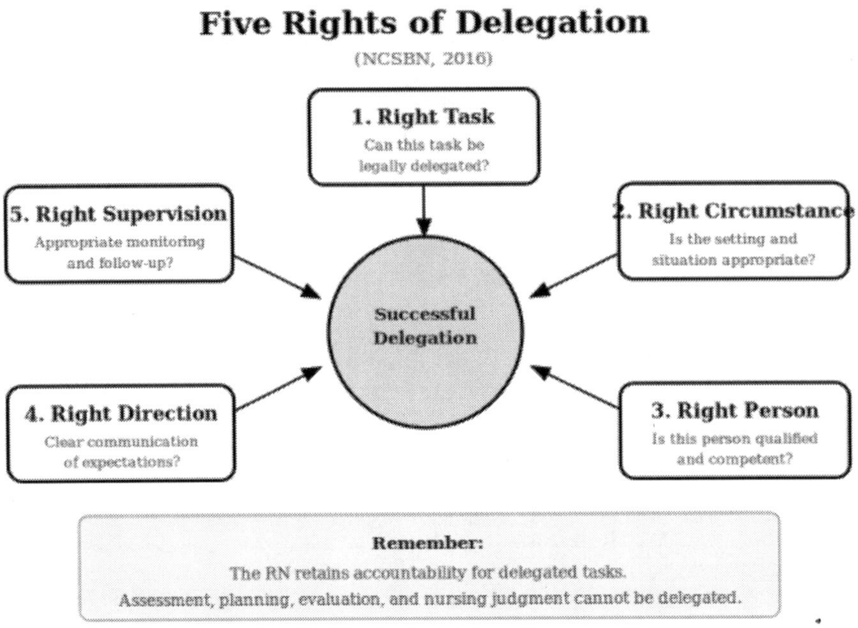

All five rights must be satisfied for appropriate delegation. The RN retains accountability.

What Cannot Be Delegated

Certain nursing responsibilities cannot be delegated to unlicensed assistive personnel (UAPs). These include:

- Initial and comprehensive assessments
- Nursing diagnosis and care planning
- Patient/family teaching that requires professional judgment
- Evaluation of patient response to interventions
- Tasks requiring nursing judgment during implementation
- Administration of most medications (varies by state)
- Any task outside the delegatee's scope or competence

Remember: You can delegate a task, but you cannot delegate your professional accountability. If a delegated task is performed incorrectly, the delegating nurse bears responsibility for the delegation decision and supervision.

6.4 Communication

Effective communication is essential to taking action. You must communicate clearly with patients, families, and healthcare team members. Poor communication is a leading cause of medical errors and adverse events.

SBAR Communication

SBAR is a structured communication framework that ensures critical information is conveyed clearly and completely, particularly when communicating with physicians or during handoffs (Institute for Healthcare Improvement, 2021). SBAR stands for:

Situation: What is happening right now? State the patient's name, your concern, and why you are calling. Example: "I'm calling about Mr. Johnson in room 412. He's developed sudden shortness of breath."

Background: What is the relevant history? Provide context including diagnosis, relevant history, and recent events. Example: "He's a 68-year-old admitted for heart failure. He was stable earlier today but received his IV Lasix about an hour ago."

Assessment: What do you think is happening? Share your clinical assessment of the situation. Example: "I'm concerned he may be developing pulmonary edema. His SpO2 dropped from 96% to 89%, and I'm hearing crackles in his bases that weren't there this morning."

Recommendation: What do you think should be done? Suggest actions or ask specific questions. Example: "I'd like to increase his oxygen and would like an order for a chest X-ray. Should I also give his PRN Lasix?"

Figure 6.3: SBAR Communication Template

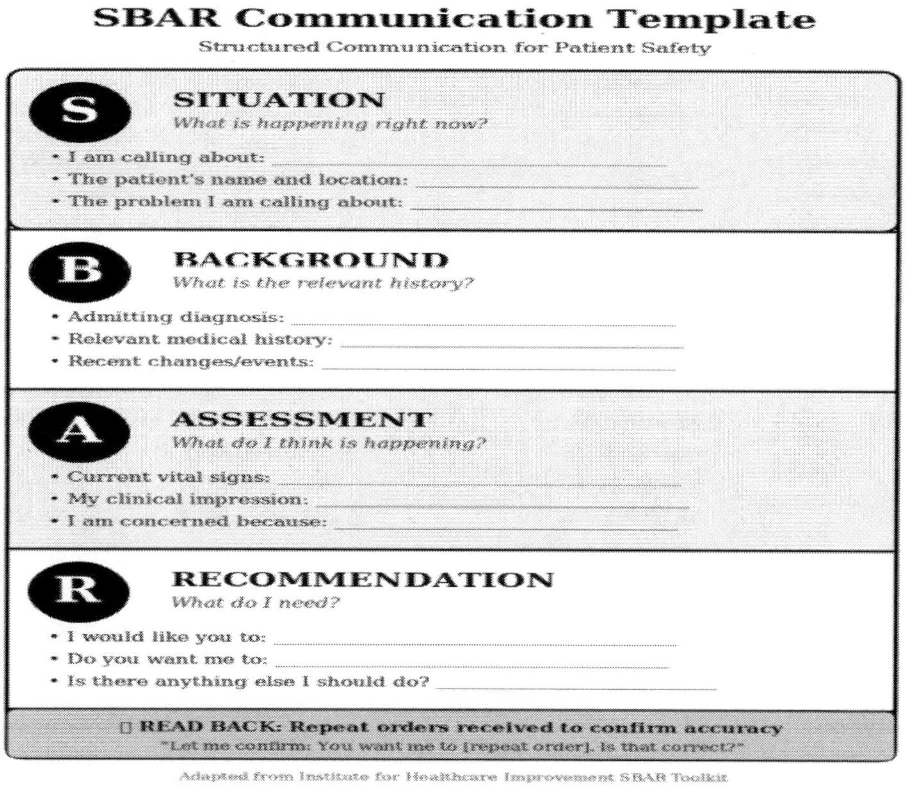
SBAR Communication Template

Structured Communication for Patient Safety

S — SITUATION
What is happening right now?
- I am calling about: ____
- The patient's name and location: ____
- The problem I am calling about: ____

B — BACKGROUND
What is the relevant history?
- Admitting diagnosis: ____
- Relevant medical history: ____
- Recent changes/events: ____

A — ASSESSMENT
What do I think is happening?
- Current vital signs: ____
- My clinical impression: ____
- I am concerned because: ____

R — RECOMMENDATION
What do I need?
- I would like you to: ____
- Do you want me to: ____
- Is there anything else I should do? ____

☐ **READ BACK: Repeat orders received to confirm accuracy**
"Let me confirm: You want me to [repeat order]. Is that correct?"

Adapted from Institute for Healthcare Improvement SBAR Toolkit

Use this template when communicating with providers about patient concerns.

Communicating with Patients and Families

When taking action, communicate with patients about what you are doing and why. This respects patient autonomy, reduces anxiety, and enables patients to participate in their care. Explain procedures before performing them, provide education as appropriate, and invite questions.

Use language the patient can understand—avoid medical jargon or explain technical terms. Confirm understanding by asking patients to repeat information back. Be honest about what to expect, including potential discomfort. Involve family members as appropriate, respecting patient preferences about information sharing.

Closed-Loop Communication

In critical situations or when delegating, use closed-loop communication to ensure messages are received correctly. The sender states information, the receiver repeats it back, and the sender confirms the repeat is correct. Example: "Give 4 mg morphine IV." "4 mg morphine IV, confirmed." "That's correct." This technique catches misunderstandings before they become errors.

6.5 Safety Considerations

Patient safety must be maintained throughout action implementation. Safety is not an afterthought—it should be integrated into every action you take.

Verification and Double-Checks

Before implementing interventions, verify that you have the right patient, the right intervention, and that conditions haven't changed since your assessment. Use two patient identifiers before any procedure or medication administration. Verify medication rights: right patient, right drug, right dose, right route, right time, right documentation, right reason, and right response.

Anticipating and Preventing Complications

Before taking action, consider what could go wrong and take steps to prevent complications. Have emergency equipment accessible when performing high-risk procedures. Know the potential adverse effects of medications you administer. Position yourself to call for help if needed. Prepare contingency plans for foreseeable complications.

Knowing When to Stop or Escalate

Sometimes the safest action is to stop and reassess. If something unexpected occurs during implementation, if the patient's condition changes, or if you become concerned about safety, it is appropriate to pause. Do not continue with an action if you are unsure it is correct. Escalate concerns to senior staff or providers when the situation exceeds your competence or authority.

6.6 Documentation

Documentation is an essential component of taking action. The medical record serves as the legal record of care, enables communication among healthcare team members, supports continuity of care, and provides data for quality improvement. The principle "if it wasn't documented, it wasn't done" reflects the legal and practical importance of complete documentation.

What to Document

Document the actions you take, including: what intervention was performed, when it was performed, the patient's response to the intervention, any complications or unexpected events, and follow-up actions taken or planned. Be specific and objective. Use standardized terminology where available.

Documentation Principles

Be timely. Document as close to the event as possible. Delayed documentation increases the risk of errors and omissions.

Be accurate. Record exactly what occurred. Do not document actions before they are completed. Never falsify documentation.

Be complete. Include all relevant information. Incomplete documentation can compromise patient care and create legal vulnerability.

Be objective. Record observations and facts, not interpretations or opinions. Use quotes for patient statements.

Be professional. Maintain a professional tone. Do not use documentation to criticize colleagues or express frustration.

6.7 Clinical Application Examples

The following examples demonstrate the "Take Action" skill in clinical practice, illustrating prioritization, delegation, communication, and safety considerations.

Example 1: Emergency Response

Scenario: While assessing a post-operative patient, you find them unresponsive with no palpable pulse and agonal breathing.

Actions:

Prioritization: Immediate activation of code team—this is an ABC emergency (no circulation).

Communication: Call for help, activate code blue, state room number clearly.

Safety: Lower bed, flat position, prepare for CPR.

Action: Begin chest compressions immediately while waiting for code team, apply AED when available.

Delegation: Direct other staff—"You, call the code. You, get the crash cart. You, clear the room."

Documentation: Time of discovery, time of code activation, interventions performed, personnel present.

Example 2: Medication Administration

Scenario: You need to administer IV push morphine 4 mg to a patient reporting 8/10 pain.

Actions:

Verification: Confirm two patient identifiers, verify order, check allergies.

Safety: Verify dosage calculation, confirm IV patency, have reversal agent (naloxone) knowledge ready.

Communication: Explain to patient what you're giving and expected effect, inform about potential side effects.

Action: Administer medication at appropriate rate, monitor patient response.

Follow-up: Reassess pain level in 15-30 minutes, monitor for adverse effects (respiratory depression, hypotension).

Documentation: Medication, dose, route, time, pre-administration assessment (pain level, VS), patient response.

Example 3: Delegating Care

Scenario: You have four patients. Patient A needs vital signs checked, Patient B needs repositioning and bed change, Patient C needs discharge teaching, and Patient D needs IV antibiotic administration. You have one CNA available to help.

Actions:

Analysis: Determine what can be delegated—VS and repositioning can go to CNA; teaching and IV medication cannot be delegated.

Direction to CNA: "Please take vital signs on Patient A first—she had low BP earlier so let me know immediately if systolic is below 100. Then reposition and change linens for Patient B."

Nurse prioritization: Administer IV antibiotic to Patient D first (time-sensitive), then provide discharge teaching to Patient C.

Supervision: Check back with CNA about vital signs, verify tasks completed appropriately.

Follow-up: Review vital signs personally, assess Patient B's skin during next rounding.

6.8 Practice Problems (20)

For each scenario, determine the appropriate actions, including prioritization, delegation decisions, communication needs, and safety considerations.

1. You are caring for four patients. Patient A is requesting pain medication (due now). Patient B is scheduled for surgery in 30 minutes and needs preoperative teaching. Patient C's IV pump alarm is sounding. Patient D's wife is at the desk asking to speak with you about his prognosis. In what order should you address these needs?

2. A physician gives you a verbal order: "Give the patient in 302 some Ativan." What actions should you take before implementing this order?

3. You need to perform a sterile dressing change on Patient A and a bed bath on Patient B. A CNA is available to help. What should you delegate, and what instructions should you provide?

4. A patient suddenly becomes unresponsive. You find no pulse. A nursing student is with you. What actions do you take, and how do you direct the student?

5. You are about to give an unfamiliar medication. The patient says, "That pill looks different than the one I usually take." What actions should you take?

6. A patient with diabetes is preparing for discharge. They need teaching about insulin administration, dietary management, and signs of hypo/hyperglycemia. Their adult child is present and asks to learn as well. How should you proceed?

7. You discover that a medication error has occurred—the previous shift gave the patient double the ordered dose of a blood pressure medication. The patient currently has BP 88/52 and reports dizziness. What actions should you take?

8. A patient's family member approaches you and says, "Dad's nurse yesterday said he'd be going home today, but no one has said anything to us." How should you handle this situation?

9. You receive an order to discontinue a patient's PCA pump and transition to oral pain medication. The patient is currently sleeping comfortably with a pain level of 2/10. When and how should you implement this transition?

10. While administering a blood transfusion, the patient reports feeling "hot" and has chills. Temperature is now 101.2°F (was 98.6°F pre-transfusion). What actions should you take and in what order?

11. You need to notify a physician about a patient's deteriorating condition at 3 AM. The patient has new confusion, increasing tachycardia, and declining blood pressure. Using SBAR, how would you structure this communication?

12. A patient scheduled for surgery tomorrow tells you, "I've changed my mind. I don't want to have the surgery." What are your actions and who needs to be notified?

13. You are giving handoff report to the oncoming nurse. What essential information must be communicated, and how should you structure the report?

14. A UAP reports that a patient's blood glucose is 42 mg/dL. The patient is drowsy but responds to voice. What actions should you take immediately?

15. You witness a coworker skip the hand hygiene step before entering a patient's room. How should you handle this situation?

16. A patient with dementia is repeatedly trying to pull out their IV and Foley catheter. The family is not present. What actions should you consider, and what interventions require orders?

17. During medication administration, you realize you've been giving Patient A's medications to Patient B for the past two days. Both patients are still in the hospital. What actions must you take?

18. A patient asks you not to tell their spouse about their cancer diagnosis. The spouse approaches you asking for an update on the test results. How do you handle this situation?

19. You are caring for a patient with a DNR order who goes into cardiac arrest. Family members present are yelling at you to "do something." What are your actions?

20. A float nurse from another unit is assigned to help on your busy shift. They are unfamiliar with the patient population and unit routines. How should you direct and supervise this nurse?

CHAPTER 7

Evaluate Outcomes

7.1 Overview

Evaluating outcomes is the sixth and final cognitive skill in the NCSBN Clinical Judgment Measurement Model (NCSBN, 2018). After taking action, you must assess whether your interventions achieved the desired effect. This evaluation closes the loop in the clinical judgment process—and often opens a new one, as evaluation frequently reveals new cues that require recognition and analysis.

Evaluation is not a one-time event that occurs only at the end of care. It is an ongoing process that occurs continuously as you monitor patient response to interventions. Effective evaluation compares actual outcomes to expected outcomes, determines whether the plan of care is working, and guides decisions about whether to continue, modify, or abandon the current approach.

This chapter will help you develop skills in systematic outcome evaluation. You will learn to establish expected outcomes, monitor patient response effectively, recognize when interventions are succeeding or failing, and make appropriate decisions about modifying the plan of care. These skills complete the clinical judgment cycle and ensure that your nursing care produces the intended results.

7.2 The Purpose of Evaluation

Evaluation serves several essential purposes in clinical practice. Understanding these purposes helps you approach evaluation with appropriate attention and rigor.

Determining Intervention Effectiveness

The primary purpose of evaluation is to determine whether your interventions worked. Did the pain medication relieve the patient's pain? Did the fluid bolus improve blood pressure? Did the teaching session increase patient understanding? Without evaluation, you cannot know whether your actions had the intended effect or whether a different approach is needed.

Effectiveness evaluation requires clear criteria for success. Before implementing an intervention, you should know what outcome you expect and how you will measure it. This clarity enables objective evaluation rather than vague impressions about whether things are "better."

Ensuring Patient Safety

Evaluation is essential for detecting adverse effects, complications, and deterioration. Interventions can have unintended consequences—medications cause side effects, procedures have complications, and patients can worsen despite treatment. Continuous evaluation allows early detection of problems, enabling timely intervention before minor issues become major ones.

Safety-focused evaluation asks not only "Did the intervention work?" but also "Did the intervention cause any harm?" Both questions are essential for comprehensive outcome assessment.

Guiding Care Plan Modifications

Evaluation results guide decisions about the ongoing plan of care. When interventions are effective, you continue the current approach. When interventions are partially effective, you may modify them. When interventions fail, you must reconsider your hypotheses and generate new solutions. Evaluation thus feeds back into earlier stages of clinical judgment, making the process cyclical rather than linear.

Supporting Communication and Continuity

Documented evaluation supports communication among healthcare team members and continuity of care across shifts and settings. When you evaluate and document patient response to interventions, you provide essential information for colleagues who will continue the patient's care. This communication prevents duplication of failed approaches and builds on successful ones.

7.3 Establishing Expected Outcomes

Effective evaluation requires knowing what you expect to happen. Expected outcomes should be established before or during intervention implementation, providing clear targets against which actual outcomes can be compared.

Characteristics of Well-Defined Outcomes

Well-defined expected outcomes share several characteristics. They should be:

Specific. The outcome should clearly describe what will be observed or measured. "Patient will feel better" is vague; "Patient will report pain less than 4/10" is specific.

Measurable. You should be able to objectively determine whether the outcome was achieved. Use quantifiable indicators when possible: vital sign values, pain scale numbers, laboratory results, functional measures.

Time-bound. The outcome should specify when it is expected to occur. "Blood pressure will improve" lacks timeframe; "Systolic blood pressure will be above 100 mmHg within 30 minutes of fluid bolus" is time-bound.

Realistic. The outcome should be achievable given the intervention and the patient's condition. Expecting complete pain resolution from a single dose of acetaminophen in a patient with severe pain is unrealistic; expecting modest improvement is realistic.

Types of Expected Outcomes

Expected outcomes vary in their timeframe and scope:

Immediate outcomes occur within minutes to hours of the intervention. Examples: pain relief after analgesic administration, blood pressure response to fluid bolus, anxiety reduction after reassurance.

Short-term outcomes occur within days. Examples: wound healing progress, infection resolution with antibiotics, mobility improvement with physical therapy.

Long-term outcomes occur over weeks to months. Examples: weight loss with dietary intervention, diabetes control with lifestyle changes, functional recovery after stroke.

Different outcomes require different evaluation timeframes. Evaluating a pain medication after 5 minutes is premature; evaluating it after 30-60 minutes is appropriate. Evaluating antibiotic effectiveness after one dose is premature; evaluating after 48-72 hours is appropriate.

7.4 Monitoring and Reassessment

Monitoring involves ongoing observation and measurement to track patient status and response to interventions. Effective monitoring detects both positive changes (improvement) and negative changes (deterioration or adverse effects).

What to Monitor

Monitoring should focus on indicators relevant to the intervention and expected outcomes. Consider:

Target indicators. What specific measures indicate whether the intervention is working? If you gave an antihypertensive, monitor blood pressure. If you implemented fall precautions, monitor for falls. If you provided diabetic teaching, assess patient knowledge.

Safety indicators. What adverse effects or complications should you watch for? Know the potential side effects of medications you administer, the complications of procedures you perform, and the warning signs of deterioration.

Trend indicators. What patterns over time indicate the overall trajectory? Single measurements provide snapshots; trends reveal whether the patient is improving, stable, or declining.

Figure 7.1: Trend Analysis Template

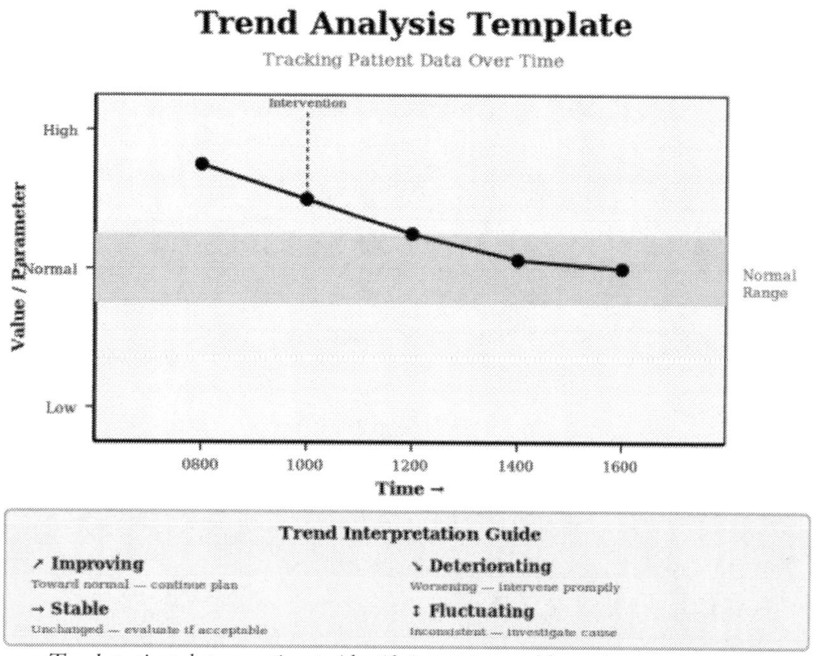

Track patient data over time to identify improving, stable, or deteriorating trends.

Timing of Reassessment

Reassessment timing should match the expected onset and duration of the intervention's effect:

- IV medications: Reassess within minutes to assess peak effect
- Oral medications: Reassess in 30-60 minutes for peak effect
- Antibiotics: Reassess in 48-72 hours for clinical improvement
- Positioning changes: Reassess immediately and at regular intervals
- Patient education: Reassess understanding immediately and retention later
- Wound care: Reassess at next dressing change or per protocol

When patient condition is unstable or interventions carry significant risk, more frequent monitoring is required. A patient receiving a new cardiac medication needs more frequent vital sign monitoring than a stable patient receiving a routine antibiotic.

Documentation of Monitoring

Document your monitoring and reassessment findings to create a clear record of patient response. Include: what you assessed, when you assessed it, what you found, and how findings compare to baseline or expected outcomes. This documentation supports continuity of care and provides legal evidence that appropriate monitoring occurred.

7.5 Comparing Actual to Expected Outcomes

The core of evaluation is comparing what actually happened to what you expected to happen. This comparison yields one of several possible conclusions.

Figure 7.2: Outcome Evaluation Decision Tree

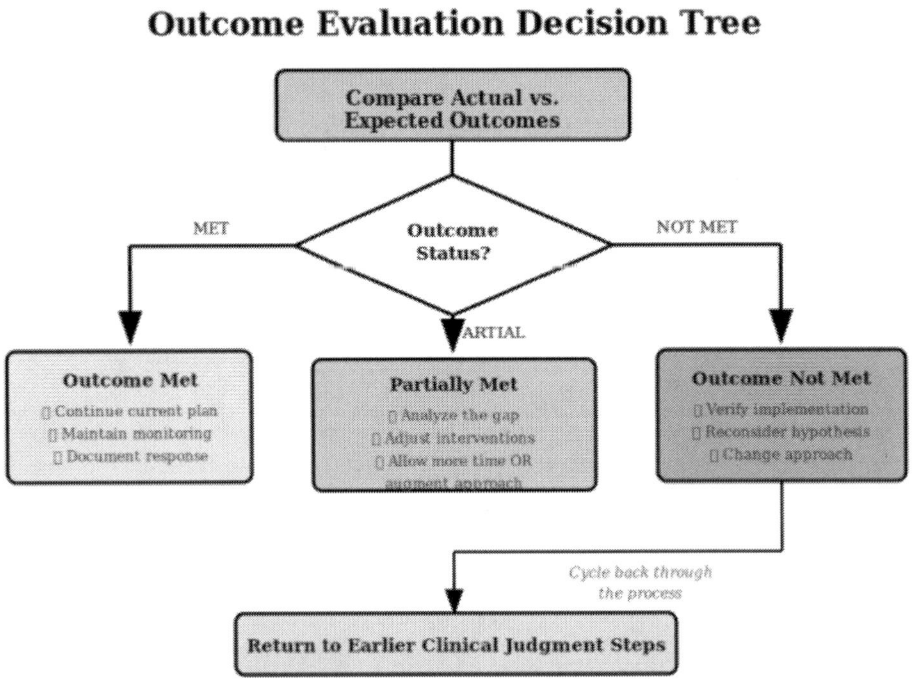

Evaluation findings guide whether to continue, adjust, or change the plan of care.

Outcome Met

When actual outcomes match or exceed expected outcomes, the intervention was successful. The patient's pain decreased to the target level, the blood pressure improved as expected, or the patient demonstrated understanding of the teaching. When outcomes are met, you continue the current plan of care and document success.

Even when outcomes are met, continue monitoring. Initial success does not guarantee continued success. Pain may return, blood pressure may drop again, and patients may forget what they learned. Ongoing evaluation ensures sustained effectiveness.

Outcome Partially Met

When actual outcomes show improvement but fall short of expected outcomes, the intervention was partially effective. The patient's pain decreased from 8/10 to 5/10 but the goal was less than 4/10. The blood pressure improved but not to the target range. The patient understood some but not all of the teaching content.

Partially met outcomes require analysis: Is the partial improvement acceptable? Is more time needed for full effect? Should the intervention be augmented, increased, or supplemented with additional measures? The answer depends on the specific situation, the significance of the gap, and the availability of alternatives.

Outcome Not Met

When actual outcomes show no improvement or worsening despite intervention, the outcome was not met. The pain medication had no effect, the fluid bolus didn't improve blood pressure, or the patient cannot demonstrate any understanding of the teaching.

Unmet outcomes demand action. First, verify that the intervention was implemented correctly—was the medication actually given? Was the IV patent? Was the teaching appropriate to the patient's level? If implementation was correct, reconsider your hypothesis—is your understanding of the problem accurate? Perhaps the pain has a different source, the hypotension has a different cause, or the patient has a learning barrier you didn't identify. Unmet outcomes often trigger a return to earlier steps in clinical judgment.

Unexpected Outcomes

Sometimes outcomes occur that you didn't anticipate—positive or negative. A medication produces unexpected improvement in an unrelated symptom. A patient develops an adverse reaction. A wound that was healing begins to deteriorate. Unexpected outcomes require rapid assessment to determine their significance and appropriate response.

Negative unexpected outcomes (adverse effects, complications, deterioration) require immediate attention. Determine the severity, notify appropriate team members, intervene as needed, and document thoroughly. These events may require incident reporting depending on severity and facility policy.

7.6 Modifying the Plan of Care

Evaluation findings guide decisions about whether and how to modify the plan of care. Modification may involve continuing, adjusting, or completely changing the current approach.

Continue Current Plan

When outcomes are met, continue the current interventions. Document success and maintain monitoring to ensure continued effectiveness. This doesn't mean the plan never changes—as patient condition evolves, the plan should evolve accordingly. But effective interventions should be continued until goals are achieved or circumstances change.

Adjust Current Interventions

When outcomes are partially met, consider adjusting the current approach. Adjustments might include:

- Increasing dose or frequency of a partially effective medication
- Adding supplementary interventions to augment the primary approach
- Allowing more time for interventions with delayed onset
- Modifying technique based on patient response
- Addressing barriers that limited effectiveness

Adjustments require clinical judgment about what changes are likely to improve outcomes. Consider what limited effectiveness and how that barrier might be overcome.

Change Approach Completely

When outcomes are not met despite adequate implementation, a completely different approach may be needed. This often requires returning to earlier stages of clinical judgment—reconsidering your analysis and hypothesis. Perhaps the problem is different than you thought, or perhaps a different solution is needed for the correctly identified problem.

Changing approaches requires humility and flexibility. It can be difficult to abandon an intervention you thought would work, but persisting with ineffective treatment does not serve the patient. Good clinical judgment means recognizing when to change course.

Escalating Care

Sometimes evaluation reveals that the patient needs a higher level of care than you can provide. Escalation might involve: notifying the physician about lack of response to treatment, requesting specialist consultation, transferring to a higher level of care (step-down to ICU), or activating rapid response. Knowing when to escalate is a critical evaluation skill—delayed escalation can have serious consequences for patients.

7.7 The Iterative Nature of Clinical Judgment

Evaluation is presented as the final step in clinical judgment, but in practice, it feeds directly back into the earlier steps, making clinical judgment a continuous cycle rather than a linear process.

Evaluation as Recognition of New Cues

When you reassess a patient after an intervention, you are engaging in cue recognition. The patient's response to treatment—whether improved, unchanged, or worsened—represents new clinical data that must be interpreted. Thus, evaluation naturally triggers a new cycle of clinical judgment.

Continuous Cycling Through the Process

Expert nurses continuously cycle through the clinical judgment process, often very rapidly. They recognize cues, analyze them, prioritize concerns, generate solutions, take action, and evaluate—then immediately begin recognizing new cues that emerged from the evaluation. This cycling continues throughout every patient encounter.

With experience, this process becomes increasingly fluid and often unconscious. What feels like "intuition" is often rapid cycling through clinical judgment steps based on extensive pattern recognition. By practicing each step deliberately now, you build the foundation for expert-level clinical judgment in the future.

7.8 Clinical Application Examples

The following examples demonstrate outcome evaluation in clinical practice, illustrating how evaluation findings guide subsequent care decisions.

Example 1: Pain Management Evaluation

Scenario: A postoperative patient reports pain of 8/10. You administer IV morphine 4 mg as ordered. Expected outcome: Pain will decrease to 4/10 or less within 15-20 minutes.

Reassessment at 20 minutes: Patient reports pain now 5/10. Vital signs stable. Patient appears more comfortable but still grimacing with movement.

Evaluation: Outcome partially met. Pain improved but did not reach target. Morphine had effect but was insufficient for complete relief.

Plan modification: Continue monitoring. Patient may request additional PRN dose per order. Consider non-pharmacological adjuncts (positioning, ice). If pattern of inadequate relief continues, discuss with provider about increasing scheduled dosing or adding multimodal approaches.

Example 2: Fluid Resuscitation Evaluation

Scenario: A patient with hypotension (BP 82/54) and tachycardia (HR 118) receives a 500 mL normal saline bolus for suspected hypovolemia. Expected outcome: Systolic BP will increase to above 90 mmHg and heart rate will decrease within 30 minutes.

Reassessment at 30 minutes: BP now 84/56, HR 120. No significant change. Urine output remains low at 10 mL/hr.

Evaluation: Outcome not met. Minimal response to fluid bolus suggests either severe volume depletion requiring more fluid, or hypotension from a cause other than hypovolemia (cardiogenic, septic, obstructive shock).

Plan modification: Notify provider immediately. May need additional fluid boluses, but lack of response should trigger reassessment of the underlying cause. Consider sepsis workup, cardiac evaluation, or other causes of shock. This patient may need vasopressor support or different intervention entirely.

Example 3: Education Effectiveness Evaluation

Scenario: You provide teaching about insulin self-injection to a newly diagnosed diabetic patient. Expected outcome: Patient will correctly demonstrate insulin injection technique before discharge.

Return demonstration: Patient correctly states dose and checks expiration date. Patient has difficulty with injection angle and does not rotate sites. Patient forgets to dispose of needle in sharps container.

Evaluation: Outcome partially met. Patient understands medication preparation but needs reinforcement on technique and safety.

Plan modification: Provide additional practice focusing on weak areas. Create visual aids for injection site rotation. Emphasize sharps safety with demonstration. Reassess before discharge. Consider diabetes educator referral for comprehensive follow-up. Ensure patient has sharps container for home.

7.9 Practice Problems (20)

For each scenario, evaluate the outcome and determine the appropriate next steps. Consider whether the outcome was met, partially met, or not met, and what modifications to the plan of care are indicated.

1. A patient with acute asthma received a nebulizer treatment 20 minutes ago. Pre-treatment: RR 28, SpO2 89%, speaking in short phrases, diffuse wheezing. Post-treatment: RR 22, SpO2 94%, speaking in full sentences, wheezing decreased. Was the expected outcome met? What should happen next?

2. A patient with heart failure was given IV furosemide 40 mg at 0800. Expected outcome: urine output >0.5 mL/kg/hr within 2 hours. At 1000: total urine output is 45 mL (patient weighs 80 kg). Evaluate this outcome and determine next steps.

3. A patient received ondansetron 4 mg IV for nausea 30 minutes ago. Patient states nausea is "a little better" but still present at 4/10 (was 7/10). Patient has not vomited. Evaluate this outcome.

4. You repositioned a patient with a Stage 1 pressure injury every 2 hours as planned. After 3 days of this intervention, the reddened area has progressed to a Stage 2 with skin breakdown. Evaluate this outcome and determine next steps.

5. A patient with anxiety was given lorazepam 0.5 mg PO one hour ago. Patient reports feeling calmer but is now very drowsy and has slurred speech. Blood pressure has dropped from 118/72 to 96/58. Evaluate this outcome.

6. A patient with pneumonia has been on IV antibiotics for 72 hours. Admission: T 102.8°F, WBC 18,400, SpO2 90% on 4L. Today: T 99.2°F, WBC 12,200, SpO2 95% on 2L, patient reports feeling "much better." Evaluate this outcome.

7. A patient with hyperkalemia (K+ 6.4) received Kayexalate and insulin/glucose 4 hours ago. Repeat potassium is 6.2. ECG continues to show peaked T waves. Evaluate this outcome and determine next steps.

8. A patient with severe COPD was started on BiPAP 3 hours ago for acute respiratory failure. ABG before BiPAP: pH 7.28, PaCO2 68, PaO2 52. ABG now: pH 7.34, PaCO2 54, PaO2 72. Patient is more alert and work of breathing has decreased. Evaluate this outcome.

9. A postoperative patient was encouraged to use incentive spirometry every hour while awake to prevent atelectasis. On day 2, chest X-ray shows developing atelectasis in the right lower lobe. Patient admits they "forgot" to use the device most of the time. Evaluate this outcome.

10. A patient with a wound infection has been receiving wound care with wet-to-dry dressing changes. After one week, the wound shows no improvement: same size, same moderate purulent drainage, wound edges still inflamed. Evaluate this outcome and determine next steps.

11. A patient was started on warfarin for atrial fibrillation. After 5 days, INR is 1.3 (goal 2-3). Patient reports taking the medication as prescribed and has not changed diet. Evaluate this outcome.

12. A patient with diabetes received education about carbohydrate counting. When asked to identify carbohydrate content of sample foods, patient correctly identifies 8 out of 10 items. Evaluate this outcome.

13. A patient with depression was started on sertraline 2 weeks ago. Patient reports no improvement in mood and continues to have difficulty sleeping and poor appetite. Patient denies suicidal ideation. Evaluate this outcome.

14. A patient with acute pain from a kidney stone received ketorolac 30 mg IV. One hour later, patient reports pain decreased from 10/10 to 8/10—"It helped a tiny bit but I'm still in agony." Evaluate this outcome.

15. A patient receiving a blood transfusion for anemia (Hgb 6.8) has completed 2 units of PRBCs. Post-transfusion hemoglobin is 8.4. Patient reports less fatigue and dizziness has resolved. Evaluate this outcome.

16. A patient with alcohol withdrawal has been receiving lorazepam per CIWA protocol for 24 hours. CIWA scores have decreased from 22 to 8. Patient is calm, no longer tremulous, and vital signs have normalized. Evaluate this outcome.

17. A patient who was NPO for 3 days post-abdominal surgery was advanced to clear liquids today. After drinking broth and juice, patient reports nausea and has one episode of vomiting. Evaluate this outcome and determine next steps.

18. A physical therapy program was implemented for a patient recovering from hip replacement. Goal: ambulate 100 feet with walker by day 3. On day 3, patient ambulates 50 feet but reports significant pain and fatigue. Evaluate this outcome.

19. A patient with a history of falls was placed on fall precautions. Three days later, the patient fell while attempting to walk to the bathroom unassisted at night. No injuries were sustained. Evaluate this outcome and determine next steps.

20. A patient with chronic pain was referred to a pain management specialist and started on a comprehensive pain program including medication adjustment, physical therapy, and cognitive behavioral therapy. After 8 weeks, patient reports average pain decreased from 7/10 to 4/10 and functional status improved—patient can now walk 2 blocks and sleep through the night. Evaluate this outcome.

CHAPTER 8

Integrated Case Studies

This chapter presents comprehensive case studies that integrate all six cognitive skills of the NCSBN Clinical Judgment Measurement Model. Each case study walks through a clinical scenario requiring you to apply Recognize Cues, Analyze Cues, Prioritize Hypotheses, Generate Solutions, Take Action, and Evaluate Outcomes in sequence. Work through each case completely before checking your answers in Chapter 10.

Figure 8.1: Clinical Judgment Worksheet

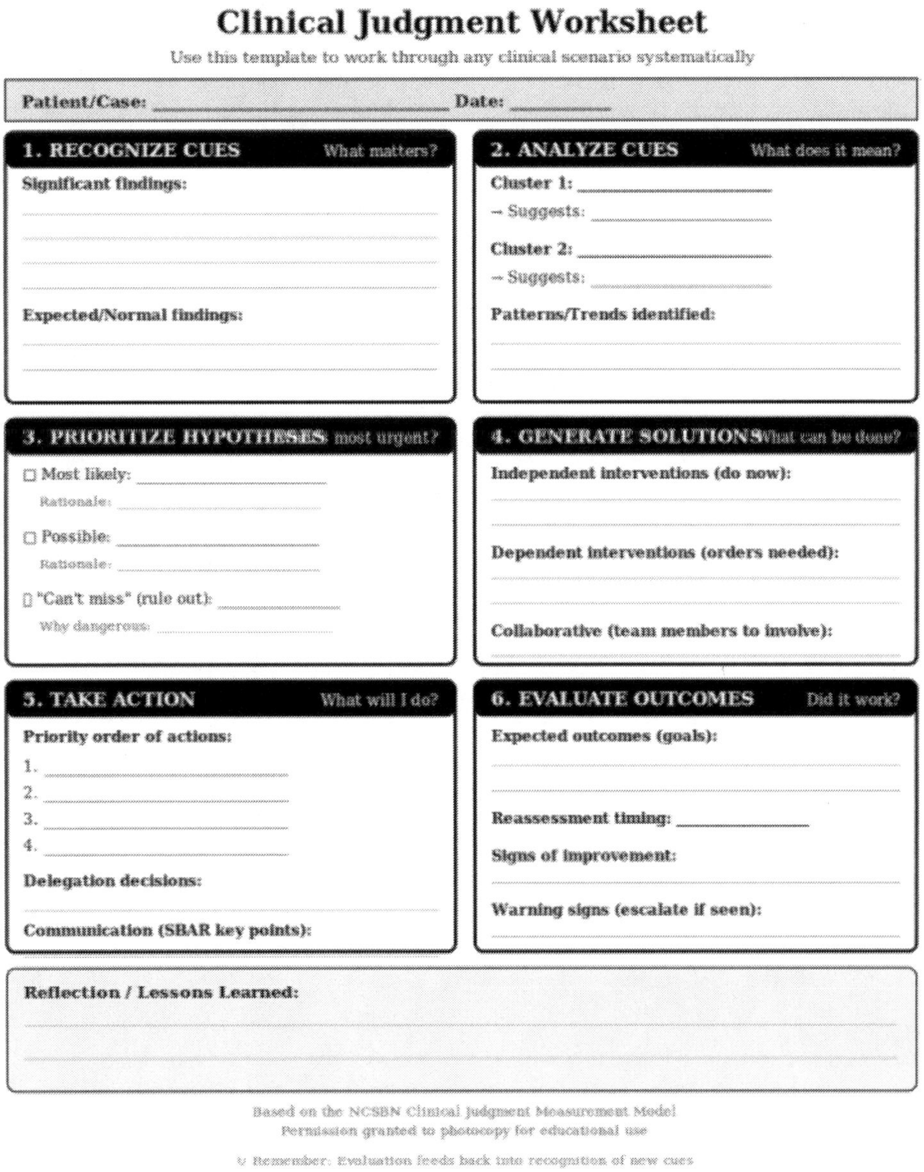
Clinical Judgment Worksheet

Use this template to work through any clinical scenario systematically

Patient/Case: ____________ **Date:** ______

1. RECOGNIZE CUES What matters?

Significant findings:

Expected/Normal findings:

2. ANALYZE CUES What does it mean?

Cluster 1: ______

→ Suggests: ______

Cluster 2: ______

→ Suggests: ______

Patterns/Trends identified:

3. PRIORITIZE HYPOTHESES most urgent?

☐ Most likely: ______

Rationale: ______

☐ Possible: ______

Rationale: ______

☐ "Can't miss" (rule out): ______

Why dangerous: ______

4. GENERATE SOLUTIONS What can be done?

Independent interventions (do now):

Dependent interventions (orders needed):

Collaborative (team members to involve):

5. TAKE ACTION What will I do?

Priority order of actions:

1. ______
2. ______
3. ______
4. ______

Delegation decisions:

Communication (SBAR key points):

6. EVALUATE OUTCOMES Did it work?

Expected outcomes (goals):

Reassessment timing: ______

Signs of improvement:

Warning signs (escalate if seen):

Reflection / Lessons Learned:

Based on the NCSBN Clinical Judgment Measurement Model
Permission granted to photocopy for educational use

↻ Remember: Evaluation feeds back into recognition of new cues

Use this worksheet template to organize your thinking for each case study.

8.1 Medical-Surgical Nursing

Case Study 8.1: Mrs. Patterson — Postoperative Complications

Patient Information

Name: Margaret Patterson, 68-year-old female

Diagnosis: Postoperative day 1 following total right knee arthroplasty

Medical History: Type 2 diabetes mellitus, hypertension, osteoarthritis, BMI 32

Allergies: Penicillin (rash)

Scenario: You are the day shift nurse caring for Mrs. Patterson. During your 0800 assessment, she reports her pain as 8/10 in her right knee despite receiving hydrocodone/acetaminophen 5/325 mg at 0600. She appears restless and is reluctant to participate in physical therapy scheduled for 0900. Her surgical dressing has a small amount of serosanguineous drainage. She states, "I just don't feel right today."

Current Assessment Data

Vital Signs: T 101.2°F (38.4°C), HR 98, RR 20, BP 142/88, SpO2 96% on RA

Labs: WBC 13,200/mm³, Hgb 10.2 g/dL, Glucose 186 mg/dL, Creatinine 1.1 mg/dL

Assessment: Right knee moderate edema, warm to touch, incision intact with serosanguineous drainage, pedal pulses palpable, last void 0530 (200 mL)

EXERCISE 1 — RECOGNIZE CUES

From the assessment data, identify at least 6 clinically significant cues (findings that are abnormal or concerning).

1. ______________________________

2. ______________________________

3. ______________________________

4. ______________________________

5. ______________________________

6. ______________________________

EXERCISE 2 — ANALYZE CUES

Cluster the significant cues into related groups. What patterns emerge? What do these clusters suggest?

Cluster 1 (related findings): ______________________________

Pattern suggests: ______________________________

Cluster 2 (related findings): ______________________________

Pattern suggests: ______________________________

EXERCISE 3 — PRIORITIZE HYPOTHESES

Based on your analysis, what are the possible explanations for Mrs. Patterson's condition? Rank them by priority.

Highest priority hypothesis: ______________________________

Rationale: ______________________________

Alternative hypothesis: ______________________________

What is the most dangerous complication to rule out?

____

EXERCISE 4 — GENERATE SOLUTIONS
What interventions should you implement or request? Identify independent, dependent, and collaborative interventions.

Independent nursing interventions (what you can do now):

____

Dependent interventions (orders to request):

____

Collaborative interventions (other team members to involve):

____

EXERCISE 5 — TAKE ACTION
Prioritize your actions. What do you do first, second, third? How will you communicate with the provider?

Priority 1 action: ______________________________

Priority 2 action: ______________________________

Priority 3 action: ______________________________

SBAR communication to provider: ______________________________

EXERCISE 6 — EVALUATE OUTCOMES
What outcomes would indicate your interventions are working? What findings would indicate the patient is getting worse?

Expected positive outcomes: ______________________________

Warning signs of deterioration: ______________________________

When should you reassess? ______________________________

8.2 Pediatric Nursing

Case Study 8.2: Emma — Respiratory Distress

Patient Information

Name: Emma Rodriguez, 3-year-old female

Chief Complaint: "Breathing hard" and cough for 2 days

Medical History: History of asthma (uses albuterol PRN), up-to-date immunizations

Allergies: None known

Scenario: Emma is brought to the pediatric emergency department by her mother at 2200. Her mother reports Emma has had a "barking" cough and difficulty breathing that started suddenly tonight. She had a mild cold for the past 2 days. She woke up from sleep with the cough and respiratory distress. Mother is tearful and anxious. She gave Emma her albuterol inhaler at home but it "didn't help."

Current Assessment Data

Vital Signs: T 100.4°F (38°C), HR 142, RR 36, BP 98/62, SpO2 91% on RA

General: Alert but anxious, sitting upright, clinging to mother

Respiratory: Inspiratory stridor at rest, barking cough, moderate intercostal retractions, nasal flaring, no wheezing

Skin: Pale, no cyanosis

Behavior: Crying intermittently, able to be consoled by mother

EXERCISE 1 — RECOGNIZE CUES

Identify the significant cues from Emma's presentation. Which findings indicate the severity of her respiratory distress?

Significant cues: ____

Severity indicators: ____

What does the "barking cough" suggest?

____

EXERCISE 2 — ANALYZE CUES

What pattern do these findings represent? How do you differentiate this condition from asthma exacerbation?

Pattern analysis: ____

Why did albuterol not help? ____

What is the location of airway obstruction?

____

EXERCISE 3 — PRIORITIZE HYPOTHESES

What is the most likely diagnosis? What other conditions must be ruled out?

Most likely diagnosis: ____

Conditions to rule out: ____

What would make you concerned for epiglottitis?

____

EXERCISE 4 — GENERATE SOLUTIONS

What treatments are indicated for this condition? What independent nursing interventions can help?

Medication interventions expected: ____

Nursing comfort measures: ____

Environmental interventions: ____

EXERCISE 5 — TAKE ACTION
How do you prioritize care for Emma? How do you support the anxious mother?

Immediate priority actions: ____

Communication with mother: ____

What should you avoid doing? ____

EXERCISE 6 — EVALUATE OUTCOMES
What indicates improvement? What indicates worsening requiring escalation?

Signs of improvement: ____

Signs requiring escalation: ____

Discharge teaching for parents: ____

8.3 Maternal-Newborn Nursing

Case Study 8.3: Mrs. Williams — Postpartum Hemorrhage

Patient Information

Name: Jasmine Williams, 32-year-old female, G3P3

Delivery: Vaginal delivery of 8 lb 12 oz male infant 2 hours ago

Obstetric History: Prolonged second stage of labor (3 hours), Pitocin augmentation, epidural anesthesia

Medical History: No chronic conditions, previous deliveries uncomplicated

Scenario: You receive Mrs. Williams on the postpartum unit from labor and delivery. During your admission assessment at 2 hours postpartum, you note she has saturated two peri-pads in the past hour. She reports feeling "lightheaded" when sitting up and says she is "really tired." She is attempting to breastfeed but is having difficulty focusing.

Current Assessment Data

Vital Signs: T 98.4°F, HR 118, RR 22, BP 94/58 (baseline in labor was 118/72), SpO2 98%

Fundus: Boggy, 2 cm above umbilicus, displaced to the right

Lochia: Rubra, heavy flow with several small clots, saturating pad in 30 minutes

Bladder: Palpable above symphysis

Skin: Pale, cool, diaphoretic

Labs from delivery: Hgb 11.2 g/dL (prenatal was 12.8 g/dL)

EXERCISE 1 — RECOGNIZE CUES
Identify the cues that indicate this is not normal postpartum bleeding. What symptoms suggest hemodynamic instability?

Abnormal postpartum bleeding cues:

____

Signs of hemodynamic instability: ____

Risk factors for hemorrhage: ____

EXERCISE 2 — ANALYZE CUES
What is causing the hemorrhage? How do the fundal assessment findings relate to the bleeding?

Likely cause of hemorrhage: ____

Why is the fundus boggy and above umbilicus?

____

Significance of fundal displacement to the right:

____

EXERCISE 3 — PRIORITIZE HYPOTHESES
What are the "Four T's" of postpartum hemorrhage? Which is most likely in this case?

Four T's: ____

Most likely cause in this case: ____

What must be ruled out? ____

EXERCISE 4 — GENERATE SOLUTIONS
What are the priority interventions for postpartum hemorrhage from uterine atony?

Immediate nursing interventions: ____

Medications for uterine atony: ____

What intervention addresses the displaced fundus?

____

EXERCISE 5 — TAKE ACTION
What is your sequence of actions? When do you call for help?

First action: ____

Simultaneous actions (call for help, interventions):

____

How do you monitor blood loss quantitatively?

____

EXERCISE 6 — EVALUATE OUTCOMES
What indicates the hemorrhage is resolving? What indicates need for escalation?

Signs of improvement: ____

Signs requiring escalation (OR, blood products):

____

What ongoing monitoring is needed?

____

8.4 Mental Health Nursing

Case Study 8.4: Mr. Thomas — Suicide Risk Assessment

Patient Information

Name: David Thomas, 45-year-old male

Admission: Brought to ED by wife after she found him in the garage with the car running

Psychiatric History: Major depressive disorder diagnosed 5 years ago, previous psychiatric hospitalization 2 years ago

Current Medications: Sertraline 100 mg daily (reports "I stopped taking it a few weeks ago")

Scenario: Mr. Thomas is admitted to the inpatient psychiatric unit after medical clearance in the ED. During your admission assessment, he is cooperative but speaks in a flat tone with minimal eye contact. He states, "I just wanted the pain to stop. I'm such a burden to everyone." His wife reports he lost his job 3 months ago and has been increasingly withdrawn, sleeping most of the day, and not eating well. She found a note on his desk this morning.

Current Assessment Data

Mental Status: Alert and oriented, flat affect, poor eye contact, psychomotor retardation

Mood: "Empty, hopeless"

Thought content: Passive death wish present, denies current active plan, states "I don't know if I could do it again"

Sleep: Sleeping 14-16 hours/day

Appetite: Lost 15 pounds in past month

Social: Recent job loss, increasing social isolation, financial stressors

EXERCISE 1 — RECOGNIZE CUES
Identify cues that indicate suicide risk factors. What protective factors, if any, are present?

Suicide risk factors: ____

Warning signs present: ____

Protective factors: ____

EXERCISE 2 — ANALYZE CUES
Analyze the severity of depression and level of suicide risk. What patterns indicate high risk?

Depression severity indicators: ____

Why does medication non-compliance increase risk?

____

What is the significance of the suicide note?

____

EXERCISE 3 — PRIORITIZE HYPOTHESES
What is the priority nursing diagnosis? How would you classify his current suicide risk level?

Priority nursing diagnosis: ____

Suicide risk level (low/moderate/high):

____

Rationale for risk level: ____

EXERCISE 4 — GENERATE SOLUTIONS
What interventions ensure patient safety? What therapeutic interventions address depression?

Safety interventions: ____

Therapeutic communication approaches:

____

Medication considerations: ____

EXERCISE 5 — TAKE ACTION
What is the observation level required? How do you create a therapeutic alliance?

Observation level and rationale: ____

Environmental safety measures: ____

Building therapeutic relationship: ____

EXERCISE 6 — EVALUATE OUTCOMES
What indicates improvement in suicide risk? What indicates increased risk?

Signs of decreased suicide risk: ____

Warning signs of increased risk: ____

Discharge planning considerations: ____

8.5 Critical Care Nursing

Case Study 8.5: Mr. Jackson — Septic Shock

Patient Information

Name: Robert Jackson, 72-year-old male

Admission: Transferred from medical floor to ICU for worsening condition

Medical History: Type 2 diabetes, COPD, recent UTI treated with oral antibiotics as outpatient

Original Admission: Admitted to medical floor 8 hours ago for "weakness and confusion"

Scenario: Mr. Jackson was admitted to the medical floor this morning for evaluation of weakness and confusion. His family reported he "hasn't been himself" for 2 days. He was started on IV antibiotics for presumed UTI. You are the ICU nurse receiving him after rapid response was called for hypotension unresponsive to fluid boluses on the floor. He has received 2 liters of normal saline with minimal improvement.

Current Assessment Data

Vital Signs: T 103.2°F (39.6°C), HR 128, RR 28, BP 78/48, SpO2 89% on 6L NC

Hemodynamics: MAP 58, CVP 12 (after 2L fluid)

Labs: WBC 24,800, Lactate 5.8 mmol/L, Creatinine 2.4 (baseline 1.2), Glucose 286

Mental Status: Confused, oriented to name only, lethargic but arousable

Urine: Output 20 mL over past 2 hours, cloudy, foul-smelling

Skin: Warm, flushed, mottled extremities

Blood cultures: Pending (drawn in ED this morning)

EXERCISE 1 — RECOGNIZE CUES
Identify cues that indicate sepsis and shock. What organ systems show evidence of dysfunction?

Sepsis indicators: ____

Shock indicators: ____

Evidence of organ dysfunction: ____

EXERCISE 2 — ANALYZE CUES
Analyze the hemodynamic pattern. Why didn't fluid resuscitation work? What type of shock is this?

Hemodynamic pattern: ____

Why is CVP elevated despite hypotension?

____

What does lactate level indicate? ____

EXERCISE 3 — PRIORITIZE HYPOTHESES
Confirm the diagnosis. What is the likely source of infection? What other problems need immediate attention?

Diagnosis: ____

Likely source of sepsis: ____

Priority problems to address: ____

EXERCISE 4 — GENERATE SOLUTIONS
What are the elements of sepsis bundle care? What interventions are needed for this patient?

Sepsis bundle elements: ____

Hemodynamic support needed: ____

Respiratory support needed: ____

EXERCISE 5 — TAKE ACTION
Prioritize your ICU admission actions. What monitoring is essential?

Immediate priority actions: ______________________________

Monitoring required: ______________________________

Communication with family: ______________________________

EXERCISE 6 — EVALUATE OUTCOMES
What targets indicate adequate resuscitation? What indicates treatment failure?

Resuscitation targets (MAP, lactate, urine output):
____

Signs of improvement: ______________________________

Signs of refractory shock: ______________________________

CHAPTER 9

Comprehensive Practice Sets

This chapter provides comprehensive practice sets designed to simulate the Next Generation NCLEX (NGN) testing format. Each practice set presents an unfolding clinical scenario with multiple questions that progress through the cognitive skills of clinical judgment. These questions use NGN item types including Extended Multiple Response, Drag-and-Drop, Cloze (Drop-Down), Highlight, and Matrix formats.

Work through each practice set completely before checking your answers in Chapter 10. Time yourself to build test-taking stamina—aim to complete each 6-question set in approximately 15-20 minutes.

9.1 Practice Set 1: Cardiac Emergency

Clinical Scenario
Mr. Chen, a 62-year-old male, presents to the emergency department with complaints of chest discomfort that started 45 minutes ago. He describes the sensation as "pressure" in his chest that radiates to his left arm and jaw. He appears diaphoretic and anxious. His wife reports he has been under significant work stress lately.

Medical History: Hypertension, hyperlipidemia, type 2 diabetes, former smoker (quit 5 years ago)
Current Medications: Lisinopril 20 mg daily, atorvastatin 40 mg daily, metformin 1000 mg twice daily
Vital Signs: BP 168/98, HR 102, RR 22, SpO2 94% on RA, T 98.6°F
Initial Labs: Troponin I 0.08 ng/mL (normal <0.04), BNP 385 pg/mL, Glucose 198 mg/dL

Question 9.1.1 — Recognize Cues (Extended Multiple Response)
The nurse reviews Mr. Chen's presentation. Which findings require immediate attention? Select all that apply.

□ Chest pressure radiating to left arm and jaw

□ Blood pressure 168/98 mmHg

□ History of hypertension

□ Troponin I 0.08 ng/mL

□ Diaphoresis

□ Former smoker status

□ Oxygen saturation 94%

□ Blood glucose 198 mg/dL

Question 9.1.2 — Analyze Cues (Matrix)
For each assessment finding, indicate whether it is consistent with acute coronary syndrome (ACS), not consistent with ACS, or unrelated to the current presentation.

Chest pressure with radiation: □ Consistent □ Not consistent □ Unrelated

Elevated troponin: □ Consistent □ Not consistent □ Unrelated

Diaphoresis with anxiety: □ Consistent □ Not consistent □ Unrelated

Elevated blood glucose: □ Consistent □ Not consistent □ Unrelated

Tachycardia: □ Consistent □ Not consistent □ Unrelated

Question 9.1.3 — Prioritize Hypotheses (Drop-Down Cloze)
Complete the following statement by selecting from the dropdown options.

Based on Mr. Chen's presentation, the nurse determines that the priority condition to address is [DROPDOWN 1: STEMI / NSTEMI / Unstable angina / Stable angina / Anxiety attack]. This conclusion is supported primarily by the finding of [DROPDOWN 2: elevated troponin / hypertension / tachycardia / diabetes history]. The most dangerous complication to monitor for is [DROPDOWN 3: cardiogenic shock / hyperglycemia / anxiety / hypertensive crisis].

Question 9.1.4 — Generate Solutions (Extended Multiple Response)
The provider confirms NSTEMI. Which interventions should the nurse anticipate? Select all that apply.

□ Administer aspirin 325 mg chewed

□ Apply supplemental oxygen

□ Obtain 12-lead ECG

□ Administer sublingual nitroglycerin

□ Start IV heparin infusion

□ Administer regular insulin

□ Prepare for possible cardiac catheterization

□ Obtain serial troponins

Question 9.1.5 — Take Action (Ordered Response/Drag-and-Drop)
Place the following nursing actions in the correct priority order (1 = first action).

___ Administer aspirin

___ Apply oxygen via nasal cannula

___ Obtain 12-lead ECG

___ Establish IV access

___ Administer nitroglycerin

___ Notify cardiology for catheterization

Question 9.1.6 — Evaluate Outcomes (Matrix)
Two hours after treatment initiation, reassess Mr. Chen. For each finding, indicate whether it suggests improvement, no change, or deterioration.

Chest pain now 2/10 (was 8/10): □ Improvement □ No change □ Deterioration

BP 142/86 (was 168/98): □ Improvement □ No change □ Deterioration

Troponin I 0.42 ng/mL (was 0.08): □ Improvement □ No change □ Deterioration

No longer diaphoretic: □ Improvement □ No change □ Deterioration

New onset crackles in lung bases: □ Improvement □ No change □ Deterioration

9.2 Practice Set 2: Pediatric Infection

Clinical Scenario
Aiden, a 4-year-old boy, is brought to the pediatric clinic by his mother. She reports he has been "not himself" for the past 24 hours with decreased appetite and activity. He attends daycare and several children in his class have been sick recently.

Medical History: Full-term birth, immunizations up to date, no chronic conditions, no allergies
Vital Signs: T 103.8°F (39.9°C), HR 132, RR 28, BP 90/58, SpO2 98% on RA
Physical Exam: Lethargic but arousable, flushed cheeks, dry mucous membranes, capillary refill 3 seconds, bilateral ear redness with bulging tympanic membranes, clear lung sounds, non-tender abdomen
Mother reports: "He's been pulling at his ears and cried when I tried to lay him down last night. He only had one wet diaper today."

Question 9.2.1 — Recognize Cues (Highlight)
Highlight the findings in the scenario that indicate Aiden may be experiencing a more serious condition than a simple ear infection.

> [Review the scenario above and identify: vital sign abnormalities, hydration concerns, perfusion indicators, and behavioral changes that suggest severity]

Question 9.2.2 — Analyze Cues (Multiple Response)
Which findings suggest Aiden may be developing dehydration? Select all that apply.

- □ Heart rate 132
- □ Temperature 103.8°F
- □ Dry mucous membranes
- □ Capillary refill 3 seconds
- □ Only one wet diaper today
- □ Bulging tympanic membranes
- □ Decreased activity

Question 9.2.3 — Prioritize Hypotheses (Drop-Down Cloze)
Complete the statement about Aiden's priority problems.

> Aiden's presentation indicates [DROPDOWN 1: acute otitis media / otitis externa / meningitis / common cold] complicated by [DROPDOWN 2: mild dehydration / severe dehydration / normal hydration]. The priority concern is [DROPDOWN 3: treating the ear infection / fluid resuscitation / pain management / fever reduction] because [DROPDOWN 4: infection won't resolve without fluids / dehydration can progress to shock / pain is causing distress / fever can cause seizures].

Question 9.2.4 — Generate Solutions (Multiple Response)
Which interventions are appropriate for Aiden? Select all that apply.

- □ Oral rehydration solution (Pedialyte)
- □ Acetaminophen for fever and pain

□ Amoxicillin for bacterial otitis media

□ Immediate IV fluid bolus

□ Hospitalization for IV antibiotics

□ Warm compress to ears for comfort

□ Lumbar puncture to rule out meningitis

□ Follow-up in 48-72 hours

Question 9.2.5 — Take Action (Ordered Response)
Prioritize the education points for Aiden's mother before discharge.

___ Signs of worsening infection (increasing fever, stiff neck, inconsolable)

___ Importance of completing full antibiotic course

___ Fever and pain management with acetaminophen

___ Pushing fluids to prevent dehydration

___ When to return for follow-up

Question 9.2.6 — Evaluate Outcomes (Matrix)
Aiden's mother calls the clinic the next day. For each finding she reports, indicate whether it suggests the treatment is working, needs monitoring, or requires immediate evaluation.

Temperature 100.2°F this morning: □ Treatment working □ Monitor □ Immediate eval

Had 4 wet diapers yesterday: □ Treatment working □ Monitor □ Immediate eval

Still pulling at ears: □ Treatment working □ Monitor □ Immediate eval

Ate half his breakfast: □ Treatment working □ Monitor □ Immediate eval

Developed a rash after second antibiotic dose: □ Treatment working □ Monitor □ Immediate eval

9.3 Practice Set 3: Obstetric Emergency

Clinical Scenario
Mrs. Okonkwo, a 29-year-old G2P1 at 34 weeks gestation, presents to labor and delivery with complaints of severe headache and "seeing spots." She had an uncomplicated first pregnancy. She missed her last two prenatal appointments due to work conflicts.

Medical History: No chronic conditions, first pregnancy uncomplicated, SVD at term
Current Pregnancy: Routine prenatal labs normal, anatomy scan normal, BP at last visit (28 weeks) was 118/72
Current Vital Signs: BP 172/110, HR 88, RR 18, T 98.2°F
Assessment: 3+ pitting edema bilateral lower extremities and hands, facial edema noted, hyperreflexia with 2 beats of clonus
Fetal Status: FHR 145, moderate variability, no decelerations
Labs: Protein/creatinine ratio 0.42 (elevated), platelets 98,000, AST 86, ALT 92, creatinine 1.2

Question 9.3.1 — Recognize Cues (Highlight/Multiple Response)

Which findings indicate Mrs. Okonkwo has preeclampsia with severe features? Select all that apply.

□ BP 172/110

□ Severe headache

□ Visual disturbances

□ Gestational age 34 weeks

□ Elevated liver enzymes

□ Thrombocytopenia (platelets 98,000)

□ Hyperreflexia with clonus

□ FHR 145 with moderate variability

□ Proteinuria

Question 9.3.2 — Analyze Cues (Matrix)
For each finding, indicate which organ system is affected by preeclampsia.

Severe headache/visual changes: □ Neurological □ Hepatic □ Renal □ Hematologic

Elevated AST/ALT: □ Neurological □ Hepatic □ Renal □ Hematologic

Platelets 98,000: □ Neurological □ Hepatic □ Renal □ Hematologic

Proteinuria/elevated creatinine: □ Neurological □ Hepatic □ Renal □ Hematologic

Hyperreflexia with clonus: □ Neurological □ Hepatic □ Renal □ Hematologic

Question 9.3.3 — Prioritize Hypotheses (Drop-Down Cloze)
Complete the clinical reasoning statement.

Mrs. Okonkwo has [DROPDOWN 1: mild preeclampsia / preeclampsia with severe features / eclampsia / HELLP syndrome]. The most immediate threat is [DROPDOWN 2: maternal seizure / fetal distress / maternal stroke / placental abruption]. The only definitive treatment is [DROPDOWN 3: antihypertensive medication / magnesium sulfate / bed rest / delivery of the baby].

Question 9.3.4 — Generate Solutions (Multiple Response)
Which interventions should the nurse anticipate for Mrs. Okonkwo? Select all that apply.

□ Magnesium sulfate IV loading dose then maintenance

□ IV labetalol or hydralazine for BP control

□ Betamethasone for fetal lung maturity

□ Continuous fetal monitoring

□ Strict bed rest at home

□ Indwelling urinary catheter

□ Seizure precautions

□ Preparation for delivery

Question 9.3.5 — Take Action (Ordered Response)
Place Mrs. Okonkwo's initial interventions in priority order.

___ Administer magnesium sulfate

___ Initiate continuous fetal monitoring

___ Administer IV antihypertensive

___ Draw labs (CBC, CMP, LFTs, coagulation)

___ Insert Foley catheter

___ Notify neonatology of possible preterm delivery

Question 9.3.6 — Evaluate Outcomes (Matrix)
After initial treatment, evaluate Mrs. Okonkwo's response. For each finding, indicate if it represents desired outcome, expected finding, or complication.

BP now 148/92: □ Desired outcome □ Expected □ Complication

Deep tendon reflexes 2+: □ Desired outcome □ Expected □ Complication

Urine output 15 mL/hr: □ Desired outcome □ Expected □ Complication

Respiratory rate 10, patient drowsy: □ Desired outcome □ Expected □ Complication

FHR baseline 140, moderate variability: □ Desired outcome □ Expected □ Complication

9.4 Practice Set 4: Mental Health Crisis

Clinical Scenario
Ms. Rivera, a 24-year-old female, is brought to the psychiatric emergency department by her roommate. The roommate reports Ms. Rivera has not slept in 4 days, has been talking rapidly about "starting a business that will change the world," maxed out her credit cards on "investments," and was found this morning attempting to direct traffic at a busy intersection "because the drivers needed guidance."

Psychiatric History: One depressive episode 2 years ago, treated with sertraline for 6 months then discontinued
Family History: Mother with "mood problems," uncle with bipolar disorder
Substance Use: Denies alcohol or drug use; roommate confirms
Current Presentation: Pacing, talking rapidly and jumping between topics, irritable when interrupted, makes grand statements about her abilities, easily distracted, denies hallucinations
Vital Signs: BP 138/88, HR 108, RR 18, T 98.8°F

Question 9.4.1 — Recognize Cues (Multiple Response)
Which findings are characteristic of a manic episode? Select all that apply.

□ Not sleeping for 4 days

□ Rapid, pressured speech

□ Grandiose beliefs

□ Reckless financial behavior

□ Previous depressive episode

□ Irritability

□ Elevated heart rate

□ Family history of bipolar disorder

□ Easily distracted

□ Risky behavior (directing traffic)

Question 9.4.2 — Analyze Cues (Drop-Down Cloze)
Complete the analysis of Ms. Rivera's presentation.

Ms. Rivera is exhibiting classic symptoms of [DROPDOWN 1: major depression / manic episode / psychotic break / anxiety disorder]. Her previous depressive episode combined with current manic symptoms suggests [DROPDOWN 2: bipolar I disorder / bipolar II disorder / major depressive disorder / schizophrenia]. The most concerning immediate risk is [DROPDOWN 3: self-harm from depression / harm from impaired judgment / medication side effects / substance withdrawal].

Question 9.4.3 — Prioritize Hypotheses (Matrix)
For each potential concern, indicate whether it is high priority, moderate priority, or low priority for Ms. Rivera.

Safety risk from impaired judgment: □ High □ Moderate □ Low

Physical health effects of sleep deprivation: □ High □ Moderate □ Low

Financial consequences of spending: □ High □ Moderate □ Low

Risk of progression to psychosis: □ High □ Moderate □ Low

Ruling out medical causes: □ High □ Moderate □ Low

Question 9.4.4 — Generate Solutions (Multiple Response)
Which interventions are appropriate for Ms. Rivera? Select all that apply.

□ Voluntary or involuntary psychiatric admission

□ Mood stabilizer medication (lithium or valproate)

□ Antipsychotic medication for acute symptoms

□ Benzodiazepine for agitation and sleep

□ SSRI antidepressant

□ Low-stimulation environment

□ Medical workup (thyroid, toxicology)

□ Encouraging her business plans to build rapport

Question 9.4.5 — Take Action (Ordered Response)
Prioritize the nursing actions for Ms. Rivera's care.

___ Ensure safe environment

___ Establish therapeutic rapport

___ Complete medical clearance labs

___ Administer prescribed PRN medication

___ Set firm, consistent limits

___ Contact family for collateral information

Question 9.4.6 — Evaluate Outcomes (Matrix)
After 48 hours of treatment, evaluate Ms. Rivera's progress. Indicate whether each finding represents improvement, no change, or concern.

Sleeping 5 hours last night: □ Improvement □ No change □ Concern

Speech rate slowing: □ Improvement □ No change □ Concern

Still believes business idea is brilliant: □ Improvement □ No change □ Concern

Less irritable, engaging with staff: □ Improvement □ No change □ Concern

Tremor noted in hands: □ Improvement □ No change □ Concern

9.5 Practice Set 5: Respiratory Failure

Clinical Scenario
Mr. Patel, a 68-year-old male with a history of COPD, is admitted to the medical unit with acute exacerbation. He was doing well until 3 days ago when he developed increased cough and sputum production after a "cold." He has been using his rescue inhaler every 2-3 hours with minimal relief.

Medical History: COPD (FEV1 40% predicted), hypertension, former smoker (45 pack-years, quit 3 years ago)
Home Medications: Tiotropium daily, fluticasone/salmeterol BID, albuterol PRN, lisinopril 10 mg daily
Vital Signs: BP 148/92, HR 112, RR 32, SpO2 84% on room air, T 101.2°F
Physical Exam: Using accessory muscles, speaking in 2-3 word sentences, diffuse wheezing and rhonchi bilaterally, diminished breath sounds at bases, appears fatigued
ABG on 2L NC: pH 7.31, PaCO2 58, PaO2 54, HCO3 28

Question 9.5.1 — Recognize Cues (Multiple Response)
Which findings indicate Mr. Patel is in acute respiratory failure? Select all that apply.

□ SpO2 84% on room air

□ PaCO2 58 mmHg

□ pH 7.31

□ Using accessory muscles

□ Speaking in 2-3 word sentences

□ Respiratory rate 32

□ Temperature 101.2°F

□ History of COPD

Question 9.5.2 — Analyze Cues (Drop-Down Cloze)
Analyze Mr. Patel's ABG and respiratory status.

Mr. Patel's ABG shows [DROPDOWN 1: respiratory acidosis / respiratory alkalosis / metabolic acidosis / metabolic alkalosis] that is [DROPDOWN 2: acute / chronic / partially compensated / fully compensated]. The elevated HCO3 indicates [DROPDOWN 3: acute process / chronic CO2 retention / metabolic problem / lab error]. His respiratory failure is classified as [DROPDOWN 4: hypoxemic (Type 1) / hypercapnic (Type 2) / combined / neither].

Question 9.5.3 — Prioritize Hypotheses (Matrix)
For each potential cause of Mr. Patel's deterioration, indicate the likelihood.

COPD exacerbation from viral infection: □ Most likely □ Possible □ Unlikely

Bacterial pneumonia superinfection: □ Most likely □ Possible □ Unlikely

Pulmonary embolism: □ Most likely □ Possible □ Unlikely

Heart failure exacerbation: □ Most likely □ Possible □ Unlikely

Pneumothorax: □ Most likely □ Possible □ Unlikely

Question 9.5.4 — Generate Solutions (Multiple Response)
Which interventions are indicated for Mr. Patel? Select all that apply.

□ Increase oxygen to achieve SpO2 >94%

□ Titrate oxygen to target SpO2 88-92%

□ Nebulized bronchodilators

□ Systemic corticosteroids

□ Antibiotics for presumed bacterial infection

□ Non-invasive positive pressure ventilation (BiPAP)

□ Immediate intubation

□ Chest X-ray

Question 9.5.5 — Take Action (Ordered Response)
Place Mr. Patel's interventions in priority order.

___ Apply controlled oxygen therapy

___ Administer nebulized bronchodilators

___ Initiate BiPAP

___ Administer IV corticosteroids

___ Obtain chest X-ray

___ Start IV antibiotics

Question 9.5.6 — Evaluate Outcomes (Matrix)

After 2 hours on BiPAP, reassess Mr. Patel. For each finding, indicate whether it suggests improvement, no change, or deterioration.

ABG: pH 7.35, PaCO2 52, PaO2 68: □ Improvement □ No change □ Deterioration

RR 24, less accessory muscle use: □ Improvement □ No change □ Deterioration

Speaking in full sentences: □ Improvement □ No change □ Deterioration

Patient becoming drowsy, difficult to arouse: □ Improvement □ No change □ Deterioration

SpO2 91% on BiPAP: □ Improvement □ No change □ Deterioration

CHAPTER 10

Answer Key & Rationales

10.1 Overview

This chapter provides detailed answers and rationales for all practice problems and case studies. Rationales reinforce clinical reasoning, demonstrate correct thinking pathways, and highlight common errors to avoid.

10.2 Chapter 1 Answers — Foundations

1. Recognize Cues — The nurse is identifying relevant information from assessment data.

2. Analyze Cues — The nurse is clustering data and interpreting what it means.

3. Prioritize Hypotheses — The nurse is ranking possible causes by urgency.

4. Generate Solutions — The nurse is identifying appropriate interventions.

5. Take Action — The nurse is implementing the intervention.

6. Evaluate Outcomes — The nurse is assessing whether the intervention worked.

7. Recognize Cues — The nurse is identifying that the BP is abnormal.

8. Analyze Cues — The nurse is connecting multiple findings to a pattern.

9. Prioritize Hypotheses — The nurse is determining the most likely cause.

10. Generate Solutions — The nurse is planning interventions.

10.3 Chapter 2 Answers — Recognize Cues

1. Heart failure patient: Most significant cues are weight gain of 3 lbs (fluid retention), worsening edema (1+ to 2+), crackles in lung bases (pulmonary congestion), decreased SpO2 (94% to 92%), and orthopnea (inability to lie flat). Together, these indicate worsening heart failure with fluid volume overload. The pattern of multiple findings pointing to the same problem makes this clinically urgent.

2. Cellulitis patient: Most relevant: cellulitis diagnosis and IV antibiotic treatment (primary concern), diabetes history (affects healing and infection risk), sulfa allergy (critical for antibiotic selection), and temperature 99.2°F (monitor for treatment response). The vegetarian diet is less immediately relevant unless it affects medication administration.

3. Postpartum cesarean patient: Expected findings: incisional pain 6/10 (normal for POD1), firm fundus at umbilicus (appropriate involution), moderate lochia rubra (normal for day 1). Requires follow-up: difficulty urinating post-Foley removal—patient should void within 6-8 hours to prevent urinary retention. Temperature is normal.

4. Confused elderly patient: Cues suggesting delirium rather than dementia: acute onset ("fine last week"), 8 hours without voiding (possible urinary retention or UTI—common delirium trigger in elderly), and medication review needed (hydrochlorothiazide can cause electrolyte imbalances). Delirium has an acute, fluctuating course; dementia is gradual and progressive.

5. COPD patient: Knowing baseline dramatically changes interpretation. These findings (RR 24, SpO2 91%, mild accessory muscle use) would be concerning in most patients but are documented as this patient's normal. The patient's statement confirms this is baseline. Continue monitoring but no immediate intervention needed. Always establish individual baselines for chronic disease patients.

6. Pediatric asthma: Relevant cues: tachypnea (RR 32—elevated for age 4), intercostal retractions (increased work of breathing), SpO2 94% (borderline), audible wheezing (airway narrowing), upright positioning and anxiety (air hunger), and parent's observation of unusual breathing pattern. The constellation indicates moderate respiratory distress requiring treatment.

7. Alcohol withdrawal: Severity indicators: tachycardia, hypertension, tremors, diaphoresis—all signs of autonomic hyperactivity in withdrawal. Complication indicator: visual hallucinations at 36 hours suggest progression toward delirium tremens (DTs), a potentially life-threatening complication. This patient needs close monitoring and likely medication adjustment.

8. Mental health/suicide risk: Highest risk cues: active suicidal ideation with specific plan and access to means (medications at home), recent major loss (divorce), giving away possessions (preparation behavior), and severely depressed mood (3/10). This patient requires immediate safety intervention, means restriction, and likely hospitalization. Do not leave patient alone.

9. Blood transfusion reaction: Both findings require attention: temperature increase of 1.6°F and new itching could indicate transfusion reaction (febrile or allergic). Actions: stop transfusion, maintain IV access with normal saline, notify provider, recheck vital signs. Even mild symptoms can progress; early recognition is essential for patient safety.

10. Newborn assessment: Concerning findings: temperature 97.8°F (hypothermia—newborns lose heat quickly), respiratory signs (grunting, nasal flaring, RR 52) suggesting respiratory distress, mottled skin (can indicate temperature instability or perfusion issues). Blood glucose 58 is low-normal but should be monitored. This newborn needs warming measures and respiratory assessment.

11. Post-cardiac catheterization: Priority monitoring: right groin site (access site bleeding/hematoma), right pedal pulse and foot perfusion (arterial compromise from procedure), and back pain (could indicate retroperitoneal bleeding if severe or worsening). Current findings are reassuring but require ongoing monitoring per protocol. Voiding need is expected.

12. PCA patient: Most concerning: respiratory rate of 10 (respiratory depression) combined with elevated sedation score and constricted pupils (2 mm)—classic opioid effect triad. While pain is controlled and SpO2 is adequate, this patient is showing early signs of opioid overdose. Hold PCA, stimulate patient, prepare for possible naloxone administration, notify provider.

13. Diabetic with hypoglycemia symptoms: Relevant cues: morning glucose 72 (low-normal), symptomatic (shaky, sweaty—adrenergic symptoms of hypoglycemia), took usual insulin but didn't finish breakfast (insulin-food mismatch). This patient is likely hypoglycemic now despite the earlier reading. Immediate action: check current blood glucose and treat per protocol.

14. Pneumonia improvement: Improvement indicators: temperature normalized (was likely elevated), WBC trending down (15,000 to 11,000—improving infection), patient feels better (subjective improvement), cough improving, SpO2 adequate on room air. These cues indicate positive response to antibiotic therapy. Continue current treatment plan.

15. Pressure injury risk: Risk factors: non-blanchable sacral redness (Stage 1 pressure injury already present), urinary incontinence (moisture damage), Braden Score 12 (high risk—scores ≤18 indicate risk), low albumin 2.8 (malnutrition impairs healing). This patient needs immediate pressure injury prevention protocol and nutritional support.

16. Atrial fibrillation: Monitoring needed: heart rate control (88 irregular is acceptable), anticoagulation effectiveness (INR 1.2 is subtherapeutic—goal typically 2-3 for afib), and symptom management (intermittent palpitations). Patient needs INR monitoring and likely anticoagulant dose adjustment. Educate about bleeding precautions and stroke warning signs.

17. Preoperative patient: Immediate action required: patient has unanswered questions about surgery. Informed consent requires understanding; address questions or notify surgeon before proceeding. The anxiety and nausea are expected preoperative responses. NPO status and medication compliance are appropriate and reassuring.

18. Chemotherapy patient: Most concerning: WBC 1,200 (severe neutropenia) combined with temperature 99.8°F. In neutropenic patients, even low-grade fever is a medical emergency—neutropenic fever requires rapid assessment and empiric antibiotics, typically within 1 hour. The absence of obvious infection source is expected; neutropenic patients cannot mount normal inflammatory response.

19. Home health medication management: Problem indicators: missed doses in pillbox, expired medications (safety risk and possible non-adherence), confusion about medication regimen, and living alone (no supervision). This patient needs medication reconciliation, simplified regimen if possible, pill organizer teaching, and possibly home health aide or family involvement.

20. Thunderclap headache: This is a medical emergency. The constellation of sudden-onset severe headache ("worst of my life"), neck stiffness (meningeal irritation), photophobia, and hypertension strongly suggests subarachnoid hemorrhage until proven otherwise. Immediate actions: keep patient calm, maintain airway, emergency notification, prepare for rapid transfer to CT. Time is critical.

10.4 Chapter 3 Answers — Analyze Cues

1. Sepsis pattern: This cluster shows classic sepsis/septic shock. Findings group into: infection indicators (fever 102.8°F, WBC 22,000), hemodynamic instability (HR 112, BP 88/54), tissue hypoperfusion (lactate 4.1, decreased urine output, confusion). The elevated lactate and hypotension indicate progression to septic shock. This requires immediate intervention: fluid resuscitation, blood cultures, broad-spectrum antibiotics, possible vasopressors.

2. Postpartum hemorrhage: The pattern indicates postpartum hemorrhage due to uterine atony. Cluster: boggy fundus above umbilicus (uterus not contracting properly), excessive bleeding (saturating pad/hour), and signs of hypovolemia (tachycardia, hypotension, dizziness).

The boggy fundus is the cause; the bleeding is the result. Immediate interventions: fundal massage, notify provider, prepare for uterotonics, possible blood transfusion.

3. Severe hypoglycemia: Analysis shows hypoglycemic emergency. Cluster: critically low glucose (52 mg/dL), adrenergic symptoms (cool/clammy skin, tachycardia), neuroglycopenic symptoms (confusion, combativeness), and context (insulin given without adequate food intake). The 6-hour gap since eating plus usual insulin created insulin-food mismatch. Requires immediate glucose replacement—oral if patient can swallow safely, IV dextrose or glucagon if not.

4. Urinary tract infection causing delirium: Pattern shows UTI as likely cause of new confusion in elderly patient. Cluster: delirium indicators (new confusion in previously oriented patient) plus infection indicators (low-grade fever, elevated WBC, cloudy/foul urine). UTI is a common cause of acute confusion in elderly patients. Recent antibiotic use may have allowed resistant organism to emerge. Urinalysis and culture needed, likely new antibiotic course required.

5. Acute COPD exacerbation: Pattern shows respiratory failure in COPD patient. Cluster: inadequate oxygenation (SpO2 88%), increased work of breathing (accessory muscles, short sentences), airway obstruction (diffuse wheezing), and inadequate treatment (no rescue inhaler). The lack of bronchodilator use explains the acute worsening. Immediate needs: bronchodilator administration, oxygen titrated carefully (COPD patients may have hypoxic drive), possible steroids, monitoring for further deterioration.

6. Femoral artery complications: Two concurrent problems: active bleeding at access site (expanding hematoma) AND possible arterial occlusion/compromise (cool leg, diminished pulse). The hemodynamic changes (tachycardia, hypotension) indicate significant blood loss. This is an emergency requiring: direct pressure to groin, IV fluid resuscitation, immediate vascular surgery consult, prepare for possible return to cath lab or OR.

7. Acute hemolytic transfusion reaction: This is a life-threatening transfusion reaction. Classic cluster: back/flank pain (hemolysis causing kidney involvement), fever, hemodynamic instability (tachycardia, hypotension), and dark urine (hemoglobinuria from red cell destruction). STOP TRANSFUSION IMMEDIATELY. Maintain IV access with normal saline. Notify provider and blood bank. Send blood samples for direct Coombs test, recheck type and crossmatch. Support blood pressure, monitor for DIC and renal failure.

8. Hepatic encephalopathy with decompensation: Pattern shows worsening liver failure with hepatic encephalopathy. Cluster: ascites worsening (increased abdominal girth), encephalopathy (new confusion, asterixis—flapping tremor), and abnormal liver function markers (elevated ammonia, bilirubin, INR). The ammonia level correlates with encephalopathy. Treatment: lactulose to reduce ammonia, possible rifaximin, protein restriction if severe, evaluate for precipitating cause (infection, GI bleed, medication).

9. Hypocalcemia post-thyroidectomy: Classic post-thyroidectomy complication: hypoparathyroidism causing hypocalcemia. Cluster: neuromuscular irritability (perioral/fingertip numbness and tingling), positive Chvostek's sign (facial twitching when nerve tapped), positive Trousseau's sign (carpal spasm with BP cuff inflation). These are pathognomonic for hypocalcemia. Parathyroid glands may have been damaged or removed during surgery. Confirm with calcium level; treat with IV calcium gluconate if symptomatic or severely low.

10. Hemorrhagic/hypovolemic shock: Trend analysis reveals progressive shock. Pattern of compensated shock progressing to decompensated: early compensation (rising HR to maintain perfusion), followed by failing compensation (dropping BP despite increased HR), plus end-organ effects (decreased urine output, cool skin, anxiety). In trauma patient, assume bleeding until proven otherwise. This patient needs immediate volume resuscitation, blood products, identification and control of bleeding source, likely surgical intervention.

11. Resolving pneumonia: All trends are positive, indicating good response to treatment. Cluster of improvement: resolving fever (102.8°F→98.8°F), improving WBC (16,400→10,200), improving oxygenation (now on room air), decreasing symptoms (less cough, better appetite). This pattern indicates appropriate antibiotic coverage and expected recovery. Continue current treatment plan, prepare for discharge planning.

12. Heparin over-anticoagulation: Pattern shows excessive anticoagulation with active bleeding. Cluster: supratherapeutic aPTT (98, goal 60-80), multiple bleeding manifestations (bruising, hematuria, epistaxis). Patient is at high risk for serious hemorrhage. Actions: hold heparin infusion, notify provider, may need protamine sulfate for reversal, monitor for signs of more serious bleeding (intracranial, GI, retroperitoneal), recheck aPTT after intervention.

13. Breastfeeding difficulty with pathologic jaundice: Concerning pattern of inadequate intake and hyperbilirubinemia. Cluster: excessive weight loss (12% exceeds 7-10% threshold), adequate wet diapers (reassuring for hydration but not feeding adequacy), significant jaundice (bilirubin 16 is elevated for day 3), feeding difficulty reported. This is likely breastfeeding jaundice from inadequate caloric intake. Needs: lactation support, possible supplementation, phototherapy evaluation based on bilirubin/age nomogram, close follow-up.

14. Atrial fibrillation with rapid ventricular response: Pattern shows new-onset afib with inadequate rate control causing symptoms. Cluster: tachycardia (HR 142 compromises ventricular filling time), symptoms of decreased cardiac output (palpitations, mild chest discomfort, dyspnea, lower BP). The rapid rate is preventing adequate diastolic filling. Needs rate control (beta-blocker or calcium channel blocker), evaluation for underlying cause, anticoagulation consideration for stroke prevention.

15. Hospital-acquired pneumonia: Pattern suggests new pneumonia developing during hospitalization. Cluster: new respiratory infection signs (fever, productive cough, localized crackles, elevated WBC, hypoxia) developing in patient with risk factors (prolonged hospitalization, immobility). This is likely hospital-acquired pneumonia (HAP). Different pathogen profile than community-acquired; needs appropriate antibiotic coverage, sputum culture, chest X-ray, incentive spirometry, mobility promotion.

16. SSRI-induced mania/bipolar unmasking: Pattern shows manic episode, possibly triggered by antidepressant. Cluster of mania symptoms: decreased sleep need, agitation, pressured speech, grandiosity ("feeling better than ever"), impulsive behavior (financial decisions). This pattern suggests the SSRI may have triggered mania in a patient with undiagnosed bipolar disorder. Requires urgent psychiatric evaluation, likely discontinuation of SSRI, possible mood stabilizer, safety assessment for impulsive/risky behaviors.

17. Pulmonary embolism: Classic PE presentation with risk factors. Cluster: sudden cardiopulmonary symptoms (chest pain, dyspnea, tachycardia, tachypnea, hypoxia), DVT signs (unilateral calf swelling and tenderness), and major risk factor (recent hip surgery with immobility). The clinical probability is high. This is a medical emergency. Needs: supplemental oxygen, IV access, anticoagulation if not contraindicated, CT pulmonary angiography or V/Q scan for confirmation, hemodynamic monitoring.

18. Digoxin toxicity: Classic digoxin toxicity pattern. Cluster: cardiac effects (bradycardia HR 52), GI effects (nausea), visual disturbances (yellow halos—pathognomonic), supratherapeutic drug level (2.8, therapeutic 0.8-2.0), and risk factor (hypokalemia K^+ 3.1 increases digoxin toxicity). Hold digoxin, correct potassium (low K^+ worsens toxicity), monitor cardiac rhythm for arrhythmias, may need digoxin immune fab (Digibind) if severe. Renal function should be assessed.

19. Resolving pancreatitis: Positive trend indicating recovery. Cluster of improvement: pain dramatically improved (9/10→4/10), tolerating oral intake (bowel function returning), bowel sounds present, and objective markers improving (amylase and lipase both trending down significantly). This patient is recovering well and progressing through the expected trajectory. Continue advancing diet as tolerated, monitor for any setbacks, plan for discharge with dietary counseling.

20. Severe alcohol withdrawal/impending delirium tremens: Pattern shows severe withdrawal progressing despite treatment. Cluster: perceptual disturbances (hallucinations), worsening autonomic instability (tachycardia 128, hypertension 168/102, fever, diaphoresis), and worsening neurological symptoms (tremors) despite benzodiazepines. This patient is progressing toward delirium tremens despite treatment. Needs: increased benzodiazepine dosing (may need very high doses), ICU-level monitoring, IV fluids, thiamine, electrolyte replacement, possible phenobarbital or propofol if refractory. DTs has significant mortality if untreated.

10.5 Chapter 4 Answers — Prioritize Hypotheses

1. Thunderclap headache: Priority hypotheses: (1) Subarachnoid hemorrhage—must be first priority; "worst headache of life" with sudden onset and neck stiffness is classic presentation; high mortality if missed. (2) Meningitis—neck stiffness and nausea fit; infectious cause needs urgent treatment. (3) Severe migraine—more common but diagnosis of exclusion. (4) Hypertensive emergency—elevated BP noted. Rationale: SAH is prioritized first despite not being the most common cause of severe headache because it is immediately life-threatening and highly treatable if caught early. CT head without contrast is first test; if negative, lumbar puncture needed.

2. Febrile infant with bulging fontanelle: Priority hypotheses: (1) Bacterial meningitis—highest priority; bulging fontanelle + fever + irritability is classic triad in infants; can be rapidly fatal. (2) Viral meningitis—less dangerous but presentation similar. (3) Other serious bacterial infection (UTI, bacteremia). (4) Viral illness with dehydration. Rationale: Meningitis is prioritized first because infants deteriorate quickly, and delayed treatment dramatically worsens outcomes. This infant needs immediate lumbar puncture (after stabilization), blood cultures, and empiric antibiotics without waiting for results.

3. COPD patient with dyspnea and leg swelling: Priority hypotheses: (1) COPD exacerbation with infection—increased purulent sputum, fever, and hypoxia suggest this; most probable given history. (2) Heart failure exacerbation—bilateral leg swelling raises concern; can coexist with COPD ("cor pulmonale"). (3) Pulmonary embolism—always consider in hypoxic patient; COPD can mask symptoms. (4) Pneumonia. Rationale: This patient likely has overlapping problems. COPD exacerbation is most probable, but the leg swelling warrants cardiac evaluation. PE should be considered if patient doesn't improve with COPD treatment. Treat the COPD while evaluating for cardiac component.

4. Young woman with pleuritic chest pain and PE risk factors: Priority hypotheses: (1) Pulmonary embolism—highest priority; has major risk factors (OCPs, prolonged immobility), pleuritic pain, tachycardia, tachypnea, hypoxia. (2) Pleuritis/pleurisy—can cause sharp, breathing-related pain. (3) Pneumonia—can cause pleuritic pain. (4) Musculoskeletal pain—common but diagnosis of exclusion. Rationale: PE is prioritized first despite being less common than musculoskeletal causes because it is life-threatening, this patient has significant risk factors, and clinical presentation is concerning. CT pulmonary angiogram is indicated; anticoagulation may begin empirically if suspicion is high.

5. Diabetic foot infection: Priority hypotheses: (1) Cellulitis/soft tissue infection—most likely given presentation. (2) Diabetic foot ulcer with osteomyelitis—must consider given bone proximity of ulcer; changes management significantly. (3) Necrotizing fasciitis—less likely but rapidly fatal if missed; look for pain out of proportion, crepitus, rapid spread. (4) Sepsis developing from foot source. Rationale: While simple cellulitis is most probable, osteomyelitis must be evaluated given the ulcer (MRI or bone scan). Necrotizing fasciitis must be excluded clinically—if any concern, surgical consultation is emergent. Initiate broad-spectrum antibiotics, control glucose, and assess severity.

6. Postoperative dyspnea with leg swelling: Priority hypotheses: (1) Massive pulmonary embolism—highest priority; sudden onset, hypoxia, hypotension, tachycardia, and unilateral leg swelling post-hip surgery is classic presentation; immediately life-threatening. (2) Fat embolism syndrome—can occur after long bone/joint surgery. (3) Myocardial infarction—can present atypically. (4) Pneumothorax. Rationale: PE is overwhelmingly likely given the clinical picture and risk factors. The hypotension indicates massive PE with hemodynamic compromise—this is a medical emergency. Patient needs immediate stabilization, likely CT angiography if stable enough, consideration of thrombolytics or embolectomy given shock.

7. Fatigue, cold intolerance, bradycardia: Priority hypotheses: (1) Hypothyroidism—most likely; classic presentation with weight gain, cold intolerance, constipation, dry skin, bradycardia, fatigue, periorbital edema. (2) Myxedema coma (if symptoms severe)—severe hypothyroidism is life-threatening. (3) Anemia contributing to fatigue. (4) Depression—can cause fatigue, weight change. Rationale: Hypothyroidism is the most probable diagnosis given this classic constellation. While not immediately life-threatening in most cases, severe hypothyroidism (myxedema) can be. Check TSH and free T4. The low heart rate and blood pressure warrant monitoring for cardiovascular effects.

8. Elderly man with acute hemiplegia: Priority hypotheses: (1) Ischemic stroke—highest priority; sudden onset hemiplegia with confusion and speech changes is classic; time-sensitive treatment available. (2) Hemorrhagic stroke—presents similarly; CT will differentiate; treatment differs. (3) Hypoglycemia—can mimic stroke; easily reversible; check immediately. (4) Seizure with Todd's paralysis—postictal state can cause temporary weakness. Rationale: Stroke is top priority due to time-sensitivity of treatment. "Time is brain"—thrombolytic therapy must be given within 4.5 hours of symptom onset. Immediate actions: check glucose, call stroke team, obtain CT head to differentiate ischemic from hemorrhagic. Last known well was 2 hours ago, so patient may be within treatment window.

9. Young woman with pharyngitis and lymphadenopathy: Priority hypotheses: (1) Infectious mononucleosis—most likely given age, presentation with severe pharyngitis, fatigue, lymphadenopathy; grayish exudate is characteristic. (2) Streptococcal pharyngitis—common, needs treatment to prevent rheumatic fever. (3) Peritonsillar abscess—complication if untreated strep; look for "hot potato" voice, trismus, uvular deviation. (4) Other viral pharyngitis. Rationale: Though mono is most probable, strep must be ruled out (rapid strep test) because it requires antibiotic treatment. If mono is suspected, avoid amoxicillin (causes rash in mono patients). Check for splenomegaly given mono risk, and counsel against contact sports due to splenic rupture risk.

10. Atrial fibrillation patient with acute abdomen: Priority hypotheses: (1) Acute mesenteric ischemia—highest priority; afib without anticoagulation is major risk factor for arterial embolism; sudden abdominal pain with "pain out of proportion to exam" early on is classic; rapidly fatal. (2) Small bowel obstruction—can cause similar presentation. (3) Perforated viscus—guarding suggests peritonitis. (4) Other acute abdomen (appendicitis, cholecystitis, pancreatitis). Rationale: Mesenteric ischemia must be considered first in this patient due to embolic risk from afib without anticoagulation. This is a vascular emergency with high mortality if not treated within hours. CT angiography is diagnostic test of choice; surgical consultation is urgent.

11. Epigastric pain with alcohol history: Priority hypotheses: (1) Acute pancreatitis—most likely; classic presentation with epigastric pain radiating to back, nausea/vomiting, alcohol use as trigger. (2) Peptic ulcer disease/perforation—alcohol use also a risk factor; can present similarly. (3) Acute cholecystitis—RUQ pain more typical but can be epigastric. (4) Gastritis. Rationale: Pancreatitis is most probable given classic presentation. Obtain lipase (more specific than amylase), assess severity (Ranson criteria, APACHE II), and provide supportive care. Watch for perforation signs if symptoms change. NPO status, IV fluids, pain management are initial treatments.

12. Toddler with stridor and barking cough: Priority hypotheses: (1) Croup (laryngotracheobronchitis)—most likely; classic "barking" cough, stridor, typical age group, sudden nighttime onset. (2) Foreign body aspiration—must consider in toddlers; no witnessed choking but may have been unobserved. (3) Epiglottitis—less common since Hib vaccine but still possible; look for drooling, toxic appearance, tripod positioning. (4) Bacterial tracheitis—usually post-viral, with higher fever. Rationale: Croup is most probable given the classic presentation. However, epiglottitis (if suspected) is a medical emergency—avoid examining throat as it can trigger complete obstruction. Foreign body must be ruled out with history and possibly imaging. Treat croup with corticosteroids, nebulized epinephrine if moderate-severe.

13. Neutropenic fever: Priority hypotheses: (1) Bacterial infection/sepsis—must assume until proven otherwise; neutropenic patients cannot mount normal immune response, so even minor infection can be rapidly fatal. (2) Fungal infection—risk increases with prolonged neutropenia. (3) Viral infection—less immediately dangerous but possible. (4) Drug fever—diagnosis of exclusion. Rationale: This is neutropenic fever, a medical emergency regardless of how well the patient appears. The absence of focal symptoms is expected—neutropenic patients cannot localize infection well. Start broad-spectrum antibiotics within 60 minutes of presentation, obtain cultures, monitor closely. The "source unknown" presentation is typical and should not delay treatment.

14. Progressive ascending weakness: Priority hypotheses: (1) Guillain-Barré syndrome (GBS)—highest priority; classic presentation with ascending weakness, diminished reflexes, post-infectious onset. (2) Transverse myelitis—can cause weakness but usually with sensory level and bowel/bladder involvement. (3) Myasthenia gravis—weakness but usually fluctuating, more proximal, often ocular symptoms. (4) Spinal cord compression—needs imaging to exclude. Rationale: GBS is most likely and is prioritized due to risk of respiratory failure—weakness can ascend to involve respiratory muscles. Patient needs ICU monitoring, serial pulmonary function tests (FVC), and plasma exchange or IVIG. The preceding GI illness supports post-infectious GBS etiology.

15. Painless jaundice with weight loss: Priority hypotheses: (1) Pancreatic cancer—highest probability given painless jaundice, significant weight loss, and clay-colored stools (obstructive pattern); "painless jaundice" is classic presentation of pancreatic head cancer. (2) Cholangiocarcinoma—also causes obstructive jaundice. (3) Ampullary carcinoma. (4) Common bile duct stone—but usually causes pain. Rationale: Malignancy is most likely given the painless nature and weight loss. The triad of painless jaundice, dark urine, and clay-colored stools indicates biliary obstruction. CT or MRCP for diagnosis, CA 19-9 tumor marker. Unfortunately, painless presentation often indicates advanced disease. Early referral to oncology and GI is indicated.

16. Pregnant patient with hypertension and proteinuria: Priority hypotheses: (1) Preeclampsia with severe features—highest priority; BP >160/110, proteinuria, headache, visual changes, RUQ pain (liver involvement), rapid weight gain (edema). This is severe preeclampsia. (2) HELLP syndrome—variant of severe preeclampsia with Hemolysis, Elevated Liver enzymes, Low Platelets; check labs. (3) Eclampsia if seizures occur. Rationale: This is a maternal and fetal emergency. Severe preeclampsia at 32 weeks requires: magnesium sulfate for seizure prophylaxis, antihypertensive therapy, labs including CBC/platelets/LFTs/LDH, fetal monitoring, and likely delivery depending on maternal/fetal status. The only definitive treatment is delivery.

17. Heart failure patient with pink frothy sputum: Priority hypotheses: (1) Acute pulmonary edema—highest priority; pink frothy sputum is pathognomonic; this is decompensated heart failure with fluid in alveoli. This is a medical emergency. (2) Flash pulmonary edema from acute coronary syndrome—MI can trigger acute decompensation. (3) Cardiogenic shock developing. Rationale: This patient is in acute respiratory failure from pulmonary edema. Immediate interventions: sit patient upright, high-flow oxygen (possibly BiPAP), IV furosemide, nitroglycerin if BP allows, morphine cautiously. This patient may need intubation if not rapidly improving. Evaluate for precipitating cause (MI, arrhythmia, dietary indiscretion, medication non-compliance).

18. Young woman with pelvic pain and vaginal discharge: Priority hypotheses: (1) Pelvic inflammatory disease (PID)—most likely; sexually active with new partner, lower abdominal pain, vaginal discharge, fever, tender abdomen. (2) Ectopic pregnancy—must rule out in any woman of childbearing age with pelvic pain; pregnancy test mandatory. (3) Appendicitis—can present with lower abdominal pain. (4) UTI/pyelonephritis—dysuria present but typically more flank pain. Rationale: PID is most probable, but ectopic pregnancy must be excluded first as it is immediately life-threatening. Check pregnancy test, then proceed with pelvic exam, STI testing. If PID confirmed, treat with appropriate antibiotics. Untreated PID leads to infertility and chronic pain.

19. Syncope with rapid atrial fibrillation: Priority hypotheses: (1) Syncope from rapid afib with inadequate cardiac output—most likely direct cause; rate of 150 can compromise ventricular filling. (2) New afib with underlying trigger (PE, MI, thyrotoxicosis, sepsis)—afib may be symptom not cause. (3) Tachy-brady syndrome—some patients with afib have sick sinus syndrome with bradycardia when afib terminates. (4) Structural heart disease unmasked by afib. Rationale: The immediate priority is rate control for the hemodynamically significant afib. However, must search for underlying cause of new afib—check TSH, troponin, evaluate for PE. The brief syncope suggests the arrhythmia itself caused transient hypoperfusion. Anticoagulation consideration for stroke prevention.

20. Progressive dysphagia with weight loss: Priority hypotheses: (1) Esophageal cancer—highest priority; progressive dysphagia (solids then liquids), significant weight loss, and history of GERD (risk for Barrett's esophagus → adenocarcinoma) are classic. (2) Esophageal stricture—can be benign (peptic) or malignant. (3) Achalasia—motility disorder but usually younger patients. (4) Extrinsic compression (mediastinal mass). Rationale: Malignancy is the primary concern given the progressive nature, weight loss, and risk factors. "Alarm features" (weight loss, progressive dysphagia, age >50) mandate urgent endoscopy with biopsy. The progression from solid to liquid dysphagia suggests worsening obstruction. Even if stricture is found, malignancy must be excluded.

10.6 Chapter 5 Answers — Generate Solutions

1. Heart failure with fluid overload: Priority: Reduce fluid overload and improve oxygenation. Independent: Elevate HOB to high Fowler's position, apply oxygen per protocol, strict I&O monitoring, daily weights, restrict fluids per orders, assess for orthopnea. Dependent: Request PRN diuretic (furosemide), anticipate possible diuretic dose adjustment, may need potassium supplementation with diuretics. Collaborative: Notify provider of weight gain and symptoms, dietary consult for sodium restriction education. Monitor response: urine output, weight trend, respiratory status, edema changes.

2. Delirious patient with safety risk: Priority: Ensure patient safety while addressing underlying cause. Independent: Reorient frequently, reduce environmental stimulation, ensure adequate lighting, maintain calm demeanor, keep bed in lowest position, consider 1:1 sitter, involve family for reassurance. Dependent: Review medications for delirium contributors, request workup for underlying cause (UTI, metabolic, infection), request PRN medication for severe agitation only as last resort (avoid benzodiazepines in elderly). Collaborative: Request geriatric/psychiatry consult if refractory. Patient factors: Restraints are last resort—increase agitation and complications. Address root cause, not just behavior.

3. Non-healing diabetic foot ulcer: Priority: Prevent infection progression and optimize healing. Independent: Offload pressure from affected foot, educate on glucose control importance, assess footwear and weight-bearing practices. Dependent: Request wound culture if infection suspected, anticipate antibiotic adjustment, optimize glucose control (may need insulin adjustment), request vascular studies to assess perfusion. Collaborative: Wound care specialist consult, podiatry for debridement if needed, diabetes educator for management optimization, possible vascular surgery if arterial insufficiency. Monitor: Signs of spreading infection, systemic signs of sepsis, glucose trends.

4. Urinary retention post-op: Priority: Relieve urinary retention to prevent bladder damage. Independent: Assist to bathroom or commode (position may help), provide privacy, run water, pour warm water over perineum, gentle suprapubic pressure if appropriate. Dependent: If non-invasive measures fail with 650 mL retention, straight catheterization is indicated—obtain order or use standing protocol. Consider indwelling vs. straight cath based on expected duration. Collaborative: Notify provider of retention, especially if opioids may be contributing. Patient factors: Review medications (anticholinergics, opioids), assess for BPH history in males.

5. Antibiotic reaction (mild): Priority: Assess severity and manage allergic response. Independent: Stop the infusion immediately, assess for progression to anaphylaxis (monitor airway, breathing, BP), document reaction and notify provider, keep IV access patent with NS. Dependent: Administer antihistamine (diphenhydramine) per order or protocol, may need corticosteroid for more severe reaction, request alternative antibiotic. Collaborative: Notify pharmacy to update allergy list, infectious disease may need to recommend alternatives. Critical monitoring: Any signs of airway involvement, hypotension, or worsening symptoms require emergency response.

6. Pneumonia with secretion retention: Priority: Clear secretions and improve oxygenation. Independent: Encourage coughing and deep breathing, splint incision if applicable, position for optimal drainage (elevated, turned), ensure adequate hydration to thin secretions, oral hygiene to prevent VAP. Dependent: Request nebulizer treatments (bronchodilators, mucolytics), increase oxygen as needed, request chest physiotherapy order, consider suctioning order if patient cannot clear secretions. Collaborative: Respiratory therapy for treatments and possible incentive spirometry, provider for possible bronchoscopy if severe. Monitor: SpO_2, work of breathing, sputum characteristics.

7. Fall-risk patient refusing assistance: Priority: Prevent falls while respecting patient autonomy. Independent: Educate patient about fall risk and consequences, offer compromise (use of walker, call light before getting up, bedside commode), ensure non-slip footwear, clear pathway, bed in low position, ensure call light within reach. Dependent: Request physical therapy evaluation for gait training and assistive device. Collaborative: PT for safe mobility assessment, family involvement in safety plan. Patient factors: Explore why patient refuses—embarrassment, desire for independence, denial of risk. Address underlying concerns. Document patient education and decisions.

8. Newly diagnosed cancer patient in distress: Priority: Provide emotional support and facilitate coping. Independent: Therapeutic presence—sit with patient, use active listening, validate feelings ("This is overwhelming news"), allow silence and tears, avoid platitudes. Provide tissues, privacy. Offer to contact support person. Assess for safety concerns. Dependent: PRN anxiolytic if severe anxiety impairs functioning, only after non-pharmacological support. Collaborative: Social work consult for counseling and resources, chaplain if spiritual support desired, oncology nurse navigator for education when ready. Patient factors: Don't rush information—patient indicated they can't think. Focus on emotional support first; education comes later.

9. Elevated INR without bleeding: Priority: Prevent bleeding while managing anticoagulation. Independent: Implement bleeding precautions (soft toothbrush, electric razor, avoid IM injections), assess for occult bleeding (stool guaiac, urine), educate patient about bleeding signs. Dependent: Hold warfarin per provider order, vitamin K may be ordered for very high INR, anticipate dose adjustment. Collaborative: Notify provider of INR result, pharmacy for dosing recommendations. Monitor: Signs of bleeding (bruising, petechiae, blood in urine/stool, headache), follow-up INR timing. Patient education: Dietary consistency with vitamin K foods.

10. Breastfeeding difficulties with nipple trauma: Priority: Enable continued breastfeeding while healing nipples. Independent: Assess latch technique (poor latch is #1 cause), observe feeding, educate on proper positioning (tummy-to-tummy, nose-to-nipple), apply expressed breastmilk to nipples after feeding, air dry, ensure proper bra fit. Dependent: May need prescription nipple cream if severe, evaluate for thrush if persistent. Collaborative: Lactation consultant is essential—request urgent consult. Consider nipple shields temporarily if severe pain prevents feeding. Patient factors: Assess mother's emotional state and commitment to breastfeeding. Support her goals while ensuring infant nutrition.

11. Hyperkalemia in CKD patient: Priority: Reduce potassium to prevent cardiac arrhythmia. Independent: Place on cardiac monitor, restrict dietary potassium, review medications for K+ contributors. Dependent: Anticipate orders for—Kayexalate (binds K+ in gut), insulin with glucose (shifts K+ into cells), calcium gluconate (cardiac protection if ECG changes), possible diuretic if patient makes urine. Collaborative: Notify provider urgently of K+ level, nephrology if not already involved, dietary for potassium restriction. Critical: 6.2 is significantly elevated—continuous monitoring essential. If ECG changes develop, this becomes emergent.

12. Post-MI patient with sexual activity concerns: Priority: Address patient concern to support recovery and quality of life. Independent: Create private, non-judgmental environment. Normalize the concern—this is common post-MI. Provide general education: usually safe to resume when can climb 2 flights of stairs without symptoms, avoid immediately after heavy meals or alcohol. Dependent: None needed for education. Collaborative: Offer to facilitate conversation with cardiologist, cardiac rehab program will address this. Patient factors: Patient's embarrassment suggests need for sensitivity. Written materials may be easier than verbal discussion. Ensure partner can be included in discussion if patient wishes.

13. NG tube not relieving nausea: Priority: Optimize NG decompression and relieve nausea. Independent: Verify NG placement (aspirate, auscultate), check tube patency (irrigate with NS per protocol), ensure tube is connected to suction at ordered level (usually low intermittent), assess for tube kinking or displacement. Dependent: Request antiemetic (ondansetron preferred—works on CTZ), request X-ray to verify placement if uncertain, may need tube repositioned or replaced. Collaborative: Provider notification if obstruction may be worsening. Monitor: Output amount and character, abdominal distension, bowel sounds.

14. Elderly patient discharge with mobility barriers: Priority: Ensure safe discharge with adequate support. Independent: Assess patient's understanding of limitations and willingness to accept help. Dependent: Ensure home health orders are in place, appropriate DME ordered (walker, raised toilet seat). Collaborative: Case management/social work for comprehensive discharge planning, PT/OT for home safety evaluation, possible short-term rehab placement if home unsafe. Consider: Can family install temporary ramp or stair lift? First-floor sleeping arrangement? Meal delivery services? Emergency response system? This patient may not be safe for immediate home discharge—advocate for appropriate level of care.

15. Lithium toxicity: Priority: Support patient and prevent further toxicity. Independent: Hold lithium immediately, monitor neurological status closely, strict I&O, assess hydration status. Dependent: Anticipate orders for IV fluids (enhances lithium excretion), serial lithium levels, comprehensive metabolic panel. Severe toxicity may require hemodialysis. Collaborative: Notify provider urgently, nephrology if severe, psychiatry for medication management after acute episode. Critical monitoring: Lithium toxicity can progress to seizures, cardiac arrhythmias, and death. Confusion indicates significant toxicity. Patient may need ICU level care depending on level.

16. Home oxygen with smoking household member: Priority: Ensure patient safety with oxygen while addressing fire risk. Independent: EXTENSIVE education about oxygen and fire risk—oxygen supports combustion, smoking near oxygen is life-threatening. No smoking within 10 feet of oxygen, ideally no smoking in home at all. Educate both patient and family member. Post "Oxygen in Use—No Smoking" signs. Dependent: Ensure home oxygen order includes safety education. Collaborative: Home health nursing for in-home assessment, respiratory company for setup and safety teaching, social work if smoking cessation resources needed. Consider: This is a serious safety risk. Document education thoroughly. If family cannot ensure safety, alternative living arrangement may be needed.

17. Refractory ascites with respiratory compromise: Priority: Relieve respiratory distress from tense ascites. Independent: Elevate HOB, monitor respiratory status, measure abdominal girth, strict I&O, daily weights. Dependent: Anticipate repeat paracentesis given rapid reaccumulation, diuretic adjustment (spironolactone + furosemide typical), may need albumin infusion with large volume paracentesis. Collaborative: GI/hepatology for paracentesis scheduling and consideration of TIPS procedure if refractory, dietary for sodium restriction. Longer-term considerations: Refractory ascites indicates advanced liver disease—may need transplant evaluation if appropriate candidate.

18. Anxious pediatric patient needing IV: Priority: Successfully place IV while minimizing trauma. Independent: Developmentally appropriate preparation (use simple words, therapeutic play), allow parent to stay if supportive, offer choices where possible (which arm, hold stuffed animal), use distraction (bubbles, videos, counting), apply topical anesthetic if time permits (EMLA/LMX), be honest but reassuring. Dependent: Consider anxiolytic if extreme anxiety and IV is critical. Collaborative: Child life specialist if available—experts in pediatric procedural support. Technique: Have most skilled IV starter attempt, gather all supplies first, warm extremity, consider ultrasound guidance. Limit attempts—if unsuccessful, get help.

19. Parkinson's patient with swallowing difficulty: Priority: Ensure medication administration while assessing aspiration risk. Independent: Assess swallowing systematically (can patient swallow saliva?), position upright, small sips of water to assess, consider thickened liquids if thin liquid aspiration risk. Dependent: Request pharmacy to identify which medications can be crushed or provided in liquid/ODT form (some Parkinson's meds cannot be crushed), speech therapy consult for swallowing evaluation, may need modified diet order. Collaborative: Speech therapy urgent for swallow study, pharmacy for alternative formulations, provider for possible medication route changes. Critical: Some Parkinson's medications (Sinemet CR) cannot be crushed—could cause overdose.

20. Painful pressure injury dressing changes: Priority: Achieve effective wound care while minimizing pain. Independent: Time dressing change with peak analgesic effect, use gentle technique, consider moisture balance (appropriate dressing prevents adherence), use non-adherent contact layers, provide patient control (breaks, slow pace). Dependent: Request stronger premedication or additional breakthrough dose, consider dressings that require less frequent changes (many advanced dressings last 3-7 days), topical anesthetic options. Collaborative: Wound care specialist for dressing selection that minimizes frequency, pain management consult if ongoing. Patient factors: Patient anxiety about pain can worsen experience—use relaxation techniques, offer control, build trust.

10.7 Chapter 6 Answers — Take Action

1. Prioritizing four patients: Order: (1) Patient C—IV pump alarm could indicate medication delivery issue, quick to address. (2) Patient A—pain medication is due now, patient is uncomfortable, physiological need. (3) Patient B—surgery in 30 minutes allows time for teaching but should not be delayed further. (4) Patient D—family question about prognosis is important but not urgent; acknowledge wife briefly, explain you'll return shortly to talk. Rationale: IV pump alarms can indicate patient safety issues. Pain is a priority physiological need. Preoperative teaching is time-sensitive. Family communication can wait briefly with explanation.

2. Incomplete verbal order: Actions before implementing: (1) Clarify patient identity—"the patient in 302" is not sufficient, need patient name and second identifier. (2) Clarify medication dose—"some Ativan" is not a valid order; need specific dose. (3) Clarify route—PO, IV, IM? (4) Clarify indication—why does patient need this? (5) Read back complete order for verification. (6) Document as verbal order with provider name, read-back confirmed. Never implement vague or incomplete orders—patient safety requires specificity. If provider is dismissive of your clarification requests, escalate concerns.

3. Delegating dressing change and bath: Delegation decision: The sterile dressing change cannot be delegated—it requires nursing assessment and sterile technique. The bed bath can be delegated to the CNA. Instructions to CNA: "Please give Patient B a bed bath. While you're there, observe their skin condition—let me know if you see any redness or breakdown, especially on bony prominences. Also note if the patient reports any pain or discomfort. I'll be in with Patient A doing a dressing change. Let me know when you're finished." Follow up: Check with CNA about observations, assess patient yourself during next rounds.

4. Code situation with student: Actions: (1) Confirm unresponsiveness and pulselessness. (2) Call for help—direct student: "Call a code blue, room [number], then come right back." (3) Lower bed, position patient, begin chest compressions. (4) When student returns: "Get the AED from the hallway and bring it here." or "Start breaths with the bag-mask—I'll continue compressions." (5) When code team arrives, provide brief SBAR and continue CPR until relieved. Key principles: Clear, direct instructions to student. Don't let student perform tasks beyond competency. Model appropriate emergency response. Debrief with student afterward.

5. Patient questions medication appearance: STOP. Do not administer. Actions: (1) Thank patient for alerting you—they are an important safety partner. (2) Reverify medication: check the MAR, check the original order, verify the medication package/label against the order. (3) Investigate why it looks different—generic vs. brand? Different manufacturer? Wrong medication? Different dose form? (4) If any doubt remains, contact pharmacy to verify. (5) Explain your findings to patient. This is a critical safety checkpoint—patients who know their medications are valuable resources. Never dismiss patient concerns about medication appearance.

6. Diabetes discharge teaching: Approach: (1) Confirm patient consents to family member's presence for education (privacy consideration). (2) Assess both learners' baseline knowledge, literacy, and learning preferences. (3) Use teach-back method throughout. (4) Break content into segments: insulin technique (with demonstration and return demonstration), dietary principles (involve dietary consult if available), hypoglycemia/hyperglycemia recognition and treatment. (5) Provide written materials to reinforce verbal teaching. (6) Include adult child in all teaching so they can support patient at home. (7) Document teaching provided, demonstrated understanding, and materials given. (8) Arrange follow-up resources: diabetes educator, home health if needed.

7. Medication error discovered: Immediate actions: (1) Assess patient—the hypotension and dizziness indicate adverse effect from overdose. (2) Do not leave patient. (3) Call for help, notify provider immediately. (4) Implement hypotension management: position flat, prepare for IV fluid bolus per order. (5) Increase monitoring frequency. (6) DO NOT conceal the error. Documentation and reporting: (1) Document patient's current status and interventions. (2) Complete incident/occurrence report per facility policy. (3) Notify charge nurse and supervisor. (4) Inform the patient (disclosure is both ethical and often legally required). This is a serious error requiring transparency and system review.

8. Family misinformation about discharge: Actions: (1) Acknowledge their confusion: "I understand you were expecting him to go home today. Let me find out what the current plan is." (2) Do not make promises or provide information you're unsure about. (3) Review patient's chart for discharge plans and orders. (4) Speak with the patient about their understanding. (5) Contact the provider or case manager for clarification if discharge status is unclear. (6) Return to family with accurate information. (7) If discharge is delayed, explain the reason if appropriate. Communication principle: Don't contradict colleagues, but do clarify misunderstandings. Family needs accurate, consistent information.

9. PCA to oral pain transition: Timing: Do not discontinue PCA while patient is sleeping—patient will awaken in pain. Implementation: (1) Wait until patient wakes naturally or give first oral dose before discontinuing PCA. (2) Explain transition to patient: "We're going to switch from the IV pain pump to oral medication. You'll still have good pain control." (3) Give scheduled oral pain medication. (4) Wait for oral medication to reach peak effect (30-60 minutes) before discontinuing PCA. (5) Assess pain level after transition. (6) Ensure PRN breakthrough medication is available. (7) Document transition and patient response. Key: Overlap coverage to prevent pain crisis during transition.

10. Transfusion reaction: Actions in order: (1) STOP THE TRANSFUSION IMMEDIATELY. (2) Keep IV line open with normal saline (new tubing—don't flush blood through). (3) Stay with patient, call for help. (4) Assess vital signs and respiratory status. (5) Notify physician and blood bank. (6) Check for clerical errors (patient ID band vs. blood product tag). (7) Save blood bag and tubing for blood bank investigation. (8) Draw blood samples as ordered (usually direct Coombs, repeat type and screen). (9) Document everything: time of reaction, symptoms, vital signs, actions taken. (10) Monitor closely for progression to more severe reaction. This could be febrile non-hemolytic reaction or early hemolytic reaction—treat as potentially serious until proven otherwise.

11. SBAR for deterioration: "Dr. Smith, this is [Name], RN, calling about Mr. Johnson in Room 315. SITUATION: He has new altered mental status and is becoming hemodynamically unstable. I'm concerned he's deteriorating. BACKGROUND: He's a 72-year-old admitted two days ago for pneumonia. He was improving until about two hours ago. His medical history includes diabetes and hypertension. ASSESSMENT: He was oriented x3 earlier but is now confused and only oriented to name. Heart rate has increased from 88 to 118. BP has dropped from 128/76 to 92/58. Temperature is 101.8. I'm concerned he may be developing sepsis. RECOMMENDATION: I think he needs to be evaluated urgently. I'd like to get a lactate level, blood cultures, and start IV fluids. Can you come assess him?" Have patient data in front of you before calling.

12. Patient withdrawing surgical consent: Actions: (1) Respect patient autonomy—patient has the right to refuse treatment at any time. (2) Explore reasons without being coercive: "Can you tell me more about your concerns?" (3) Address specific concerns if possible (fear, new information, financial concerns). (4) Notify surgeon immediately—they need to speak with patient. (5) Notify anesthesia and OR to potentially delay case. (6) Document patient's statement and notification of team. (7) Ensure patient understands consequences of refusing surgery (informed refusal). Do NOT pressure patient. Do NOT proceed without valid consent. If patient is competent and refuses, surgery cannot proceed regardless of medical recommendation.

13. Handoff report structure: Essential elements using I-SBAR or similar structure: INTRODUCTION: Patient name, age, room number, admitting diagnosis, physician. SITUATION: Why patient is here, current status, code status. BACKGROUND: Relevant history, allergies, current day of hospitalization. ASSESSMENT: Latest vital signs and trends, pain status, neurological status, pertinent assessment findings, key lab results. RECOMMENDATION/PLAN: What's pending (tests, consults, procedures), anticipated needs for the shift, any special considerations. Also include: IV access and fluids, diet, activity level, elimination status, safety concerns (fall risk, isolation), family situation, and what to watch for. Allow time for questions. Bedside handoff when possible for visual assessment.

14. Severe hypoglycemia: Immediate actions: (1) This is urgent—glucose 42 with drowsiness indicates severe hypoglycemia. (2) Stay with patient, call for help. (3) If patient can swallow safely, give 15-20g fast-acting carbohydrate (4 oz juice, glucose tablets). (4) If patient cannot swallow safely or loses consciousness, call for emergency assistance and prepare for IV dextrose (D50) or glucagon per protocol/orders. (5) Recheck glucose in 15 minutes. (6) Once stable, give longer-acting carbohydrate to prevent recurrence. (7) Investigate cause: missed meal, too much insulin, increased activity? (8) Notify provider. (9) Document thoroughly: initial glucose, symptoms, treatment, response, follow-up glucose. UAP did appropriate thing reporting immediately—reinforce this.

15. Hand hygiene violation: Approach: This must be addressed—patient safety is at stake—but approach professionally. Options: (1) In the moment: "Hey, I noticed you didn't grab the sanitizer. Want me to hold the door while you get some?" (non-confrontational, assumes positive intent). (2) After the fact: Private conversation—"I noticed earlier you went into Mr. Smith's room without sanitizing. I know it's easy to forget when we're busy. Just wanted to mention it." (3) If pattern continues: Report to charge nurse or supervisor. Principles: Speak up for patient safety. Assume colleagues want to do the right thing. Don't embarrass publicly. Escalate if behavior doesn't change. Hand hygiene compliance is everyone's responsibility.

16. Dementia patient removing lines: Actions without orders: Reorient gently, distraction techniques, check for discomfort or unmet needs driving behavior, hide lines under gown or sleeve, consider mittens if available without restraint order, ensure 1:1 observation if possible, involve family via phone if available. Actions requiring orders: Physical restraints (last resort, requires order and frequent monitoring), chemical restraint/sedation (rarely appropriate for this), consider whether IV and Foley are truly necessary—could patient have saline lock and void independently or with prompted toileting? Alternative considerations: Is the line causing discomfort? Is this sundowning (timing)? Could confusion be new (delirium workup)? Priority is the least restrictive intervention that maintains safety.

17. Two-day medication error: This is serious—potentially harming two patients. Immediate actions: (1) Assess both patients immediately for adverse effects. (2) Notify provider for both patients. (3) Notify charge nurse and supervisor. (4) Document current patient status for both. (5) Review what medications each patient should have received vs. what they got—assess for harm. (6) Complete incident reports for both patients. (7) Patients must be informed (disclosure). System review: How did this happen for two days? Identification process failure? What safeguards failed? This is a system issue, not just individual error. Expect investigation and process improvement. Be honest and cooperative with review.

18. Patient confidentiality with family: Actions: (1) You cannot share information without patient consent—this is a HIPAA requirement and ethical obligation. (2) To spouse: "I understand you're concerned. However, I need to respect your husband's privacy. I'd encourage you to speak with him directly about his care." (3) Do NOT confirm or deny diagnosis. Do NOT indicate that there are "results" at all. (4) Inform the patient that their spouse is asking. (5) Offer to facilitate conversation between patient and spouse if patient wishes. (6) Document that patient requested information not be shared and that you maintained confidentiality. Complex situation: This may indicate family dynamics that social work could help address, but the patient's wishes must be respected unless patient lacks capacity.

19. DNR patient in arrest: Actions: (1) Do NOT initiate CPR or other resuscitative measures—honor the DNR order. (2) Provide comfort measures: stay with patient, position for comfort, suction if needed for comfort. (3) To family: "I know this is very difficult. Your father made the decision that if his heart stopped, he did not want CPR. We are respecting his wishes and keeping him comfortable. I am so sorry." (4) Notify physician. (5) Allow family to be present. (6) Provide emotional support—this is a nursing priority. (7) Document time of death, presence of DNR, comfort measures provided. Key: DNR means Do Not Resuscitate—it does not mean Do Not Care. Comfort care continues. Family support is essential nursing role.

20. Orienting float nurse: Actions: (1) Welcome them and acknowledge adjustment: "Thanks for helping us today. I know it's an adjustment coming to a new unit." (2) Brief unit orientation: key supplies, crash cart location, code procedures, any unit-specific protocols. (3) Assess their comfort level: "What patient populations are you most comfortable with?" (4) Assign patients strategically—give them more stable patients, keep complex/high-acuity patients yourself. (5) Provide clear expectations: "Please let me know if anything concerns you. I'd rather you ask than be unsure." (6) Check in frequently. (7) Be available for questions. (8) Provide feedback at end of shift. Supervision responsibility: As the regular unit nurse, you have responsibility to ensure patients receive safe care. Don't assume expertise—verify competency.

10.8 Chapter 7 Answers — Evaluate Outcomes

1. Asthma nebulizer treatment: Outcome MET. All indicators show significant improvement: respiratory rate decreased from 28 to 22, oxygen saturation improved from 89% to 94%, ability to speak in full sentences (indicating less air trapping), and wheezing decreased. This is a good response to bronchodilator therapy. Next steps: Continue monitoring, ensure patient has PRN treatments available, consider whether scheduled treatments are needed, reinforce proper inhaler technique for maintenance, monitor for rebound bronchospasm.

2. Furosemide response: Outcome NOT MET. Expected output: >0.5 mL/kg/hr × 80 kg × 2 hours = >80 mL. Actual output: 45 mL. This is diuretic resistance, common in advanced heart failure. Next steps: Notify provider immediately. Options include: repeat or increase furosemide dose, add thiazide diuretic for synergy ("sequential nephron blockade"), assess for contributing factors (NSAIDs, hypotension limiting renal perfusion), check renal function. May need continuous furosemide infusion or ultrafiltration if refractory. This is concerning for decompensated heart failure.

3. Ondansetron for nausea: Outcome PARTIALLY MET. Nausea improved from 7/10 to 4/10 and no vomiting occurred (positive). However, nausea persists at a moderate level. Next steps: This partial response is acceptable for now—ondansetron may continue to work. Reassess in another 30 minutes. If nausea persists or worsens, consider additional or alternative antiemetics (promethazine, prochlorperazine, or different mechanism). Assess for underlying cause of nausea (medication side effect, GI issue, etc.).

4. Pressure injury progression: Outcome NOT MET—condition worsened. The intervention (repositioning) was intended to prevent progression, but the injury advanced from Stage 1 to Stage 2. Next steps: (1) Reassess contributing factors—is patient being repositioned correctly? Are there other pressure points? What is nutritional status? Is there incontinence? (2) Request wound care consult. (3) Consider pressure-redistributing surface (specialty mattress). (4) Assess for shear and friction during repositioning. (5) Optimize nutrition for wound healing. (6) Document progression and notify provider. The intervention may have been inadequate or there are contributing factors not being addressed.

5. Lorazepam adverse effects: UNEXPECTED NEGATIVE OUTCOME. While anxiety improved (intended effect), the patient is experiencing adverse effects: excessive sedation (drowsiness, slurred speech) and hypotension (significant drop from 118/72 to 96/58). This is an excessive response to the medication. Next steps: (1) Do NOT give additional doses. (2) Ensure patient safety—fall precautions, bed in low position, side rails up. (3) Monitor vital signs frequently. (4) Keep patient NPO until more alert (aspiration risk). (5) Notify provider of adverse response. (6) Document reaction thoroughly. (7) Consider whether this patient is unusually sensitive to benzodiazepines or has contributing factors (elderly, liver disease, other sedating medications). Future dosing should be reduced.

6. Pneumonia treatment response: Outcome MET. Excellent response to antibiotic therapy across multiple indicators: temperature trending down (102.8→99.2), WBC decreasing (18,400→12,200), oxygenation improving (90%→95% on less supplemental O2), and subjective improvement (patient feels better). This indicates appropriate antibiotic coverage and expected recovery trajectory. Next steps: Continue current antibiotic regimen to complete full course. Continue monitoring. Begin planning for discharge when appropriate. Consider transition from IV to oral antibiotics if continued improvement.

7. Hyperkalemia treatment: Outcome NOT MET. Potassium decreased minimally (6.4→6.2) and ECG still shows peaked T waves indicating ongoing cardiac risk. This is inadequate response to treatment. Next steps: This is urgent—patient remains at risk for cardiac arrhythmia. (1) Notify provider immediately. (2) Continuous cardiac monitoring. (3) Additional treatment options: repeat Kayexalate, additional insulin/glucose, calcium gluconate for cardiac protection (doesn't lower K+ but stabilizes cardiac membrane), consider emergent hemodialysis if patient has renal failure. (4) Reassess for ongoing sources of potassium (medications, tissue breakdown, diet).

8. BiPAP for respiratory failure: Outcome MET. Significant improvement in all ABG parameters: pH improving toward normal (7.28→7.34), CO2 decreasing (68→54), oxygenation improving (52→72). Clinical improvement correlates: patient more alert, decreased work of breathing. BiPAP is working—the patient is being effectively ventilated non-invasively. Next steps: Continue BiPAP, continue monitoring ABGs per protocol, watch for improvement that allows weaning, or deterioration that might require intubation. Patient avoided intubation, which is the goal of BiPAP in COPD exacerbation.

9. Incentive spirometry non-compliance: Outcome NOT MET due to intervention not being implemented. The intervention (incentive spirometry) was prescribed but patient didn't perform it adequately. This is an adherence issue, not an intervention failure. Next steps: (1) Educate patient about importance—explain that atelectasis developed because the exercises weren't done. (2) Assess barriers: pain with deep breathing? Doesn't understand technique? Too drowsy from medications? (3) Provide better support: set alarms, have staff prompt and supervise use, ensure pain is controlled before exercises. (4) Now need treatment for atelectasis: aggressive pulmonary toilet, possible respiratory therapy. Prevention failed; now need treatment.

10. Wound not improving: Outcome NOT MET. After one week of treatment, wound shows no improvement on any parameter. This suggests: (1) Current treatment is inadequate, (2) Underlying infection is not being addressed, or (3) Contributing factors are preventing healing. Next steps: (1) Request wound care specialist consult. (2) Obtain wound culture if not recently done—organism may be resistant. (3) Reassess antibiotic coverage. (4) Evaluate for factors impeding healing: diabetes control, nutrition, vascular status, immune function. (5) Consider different wound care approach—wet-to-dry may not be optimal for this wound. Modern wound care often uses moisture-retentive dressings instead.

11. Warfarin subtherapeutic: Outcome NOT YET MET—but this may be expected. Warfarin takes 5-7 days to reach full effect due to its mechanism (depleting clotting factors). INR of 1.3 after 5 days indicates the medication is starting to work but hasn't reached therapeutic level yet. Next steps: (1) Continue current therapy—don't assume failure yet. (2) Recheck INR in 2-3 days. (3) If still subtherapeutic after 7-10 days, dose adjustment may be needed. (4) Ensure patient continues bridging anticoagulation (if ordered) until INR therapeutic. (5) Review for drug interactions or conditions affecting warfarin metabolism. This is likely normal delayed response, not treatment failure.

12. Diabetes education: Outcome PARTIALLY MET. Patient correctly identified 8 of 10 items (80%), which demonstrates good understanding but not complete mastery. Next steps: (1) Review the 2 items patient missed—what was the confusion? (2) Provide additional teaching on those specific foods. (3) Consider whether the errors were clinically significant (would they substantially affect glucose management?). (4) Provide reference materials for home use (carb counting guide, app). (5) Reassess understanding after additional teaching. (6) Arrange follow-up with diabetes educator. 80% may be acceptable for initial teaching, but continued reinforcement is needed.

13. SSRI early evaluation: Outcome NOT YET DETERMINABLE. SSRIs typically require 4-6 weeks to reach full therapeutic effect—2 weeks is too early to evaluate effectiveness. The lack of improvement at 2 weeks is expected, not a treatment failure. Next steps: (1) Educate patient about expected timeline—improvement usually begins around weeks 3-4. (2) Ensure medication compliance. (3) Monitor for worsening depression or emergence of suicidal ideation (can occur early in treatment before mood improves). (4) Continue current regimen and reassess at 4-6 weeks. (5) Ensure patient has support and knows when to seek help if symptoms worsen. Do NOT change medication yet based on 2-week assessment.

14. Kidney stone pain: Outcome NOT MET. Pain decreased only from 10/10 to 8/10—still "agony." Ketorolac, while often effective for renal colic, was inadequate for this patient. Next steps: (1) Notify provider of inadequate response. (2) Patient needs additional analgesia—consider opioid medication for severe acute pain. (3) Combination therapy (NSAID + opioid) may be more effective than either alone. (4) Ensure patient is receiving IV fluids to promote stone passage. (5) Evaluate for complications: complete obstruction, infection (pyuria with obstruction is emergency). Pain this severe warrants aggressive management while addressing the underlying stone.

15. Blood transfusion response: Outcome MET. Hemoglobin increased appropriately (6.8→8.4, approximately 0.8 g/dL increase per unit, which is expected). Symptomatic improvement confirms clinical benefit: fatigue improved, dizziness resolved. Next steps: Continue monitoring for delayed transfusion reactions. Evaluate whether additional transfusion is needed (goal Hgb varies by patient condition). Investigate and address cause of anemia to prevent recurrence. Patient should feel significantly better with improved oxygen-carrying capacity.

16. Alcohol withdrawal treatment: Outcome MET. Excellent response to CIWA-based benzodiazepine protocol: CIWA scores decreased from 22 (severe) to 8 (mild), clinical symptoms resolved (calm, no tremors), and vital signs normalized. This indicates effective management of withdrawal. Next steps: Continue CIWA monitoring with frequency appropriate to score. Patient is now in mild withdrawal—continue protocol but anticipate decreasing benzodiazepine requirements. Watch for breakthrough symptoms. Ensure thiamine and nutritional support. Begin planning for ongoing addiction treatment and support.

17. Diet advancement intolerance: Outcome NOT MET. Patient was unable to tolerate advancement to clear liquids. Nausea and vomiting after 3 days NPO following abdominal surgery could indicate: normal slow GI recovery, ileus, or early obstruction. Next steps: (1) Return to NPO status. (2) Notify provider. (3) Assess for signs of ileus or obstruction: abdominal distension, absent bowel sounds, increasing pain. (4) May need NG tube if vomiting continues. (5) Evaluate when to retry diet advancement—usually wait 24 hours and reassess GI function. This is a setback but not uncommon post-abdominal surgery; requires careful reassessment before next attempt.

18. Physical therapy progress: Outcome PARTIALLY MET. Patient achieved 50% of goal (50 feet vs. 100 feet target) but pain and fatigue limited further progress. Next steps: (1) This is progress, though below target. (2) Evaluate barriers: Is pain adequately controlled before PT sessions? Is patient deconditioned? Are there medical complications limiting progress? (3) Ensure adequate pain medication before PT. (4) May need to adjust goal—100 feet by day 3 may have been ambitious for this patient. (5) Continue therapy with modified expectations. (6) Communicate with PT about barriers and adjusted plan. Slow progress is still progress; ensure patient isn't discouraged.

19. Fall despite precautions: Outcome NOT MET. The goal of fall precautions is to prevent falls—a fall occurred. This is a failure of the prevention strategy. However, no injury resulted, which mitigates the outcome severity. Next steps: (1) Complete post-fall assessment and documentation. (2) Incident report per facility policy. (3) Analyze why fall occurred: patient went unassisted at night—was call light used? What barriers prevented patient from calling for help? Toileting needs? (4) Modify fall prevention plan: bedside commode? More frequent toileting rounds? Bed alarm? Different room location? (5) Patient education reinforcement. The fall indicates current interventions were insufficient for this patient's risk level.

20. Chronic pain program: Outcome MET. After 8 weeks of comprehensive pain management: pain decreased from 7/10 to 4/10 (43% reduction is clinically significant for chronic pain), and functional status substantially improved (walking 2 blocks, sleeping through night are meaningful functional gains). Next steps: Continue current multimodal program. Set new functional goals now that baseline has improved. Chronic pain management is ongoing—this success represents progress, not cure. Continue all components of the program: medication, PT, CBT. Patient is responding well to comprehensive approach; this validates the multimodal strategy over single-modality treatment.

10.9 Chapter 8 Case Study Answers

Case Study 8.1 Answers — Mrs. Patterson (Postoperative Complications)

Exercise 1 — Recognize Cues: Significant cues include: (1) Temperature 101.2°F—elevated, suggests infection; (2) Pain 8/10 despite medication—uncontrolled, worsening pain; (3) WBC 13,200—elevated, immune response; (4) Blood glucose 186—elevated, stress response and poor diabetes control; (5) Patient statement "I don't feel right"—vague but significant; (6) Knee warm to touch—may indicate infection beyond expected postop inflammation; (7) Heart rate 98—mildly elevated, may indicate pain or early infection response.

Exercise 2 — Analyze Cues: Cluster 1: Fever + elevated WBC + warm knee + uncontrolled pain = infection pattern suggesting surgical site infection. Cluster 2: Elevated glucose + "not feeling right" + elevated BP = stress response indicating body fighting something. The vague symptom "doesn't feel right" is particularly significant in elderly and diabetic patients who may not mount typical inflammatory responses.

Exercise 3 — Prioritize Hypotheses: Most likely: Surgical site infection (SSI)—fever, elevated WBC, uncontrolled pain, warmth at surgical site. Alternative: DVT (recent surgery is risk factor, but no calf findings noted). Must rule out: Sepsis—if SSI is present and untreated, can progress rapidly, especially in diabetic patient.

Exercise 4 — Generate Solutions: Independent: Assess surgical site closely, check for increased drainage/redness/purulence, keep patient comfortable, monitor vital signs more frequently. Dependent: Request provider evaluation, anticipate orders for wound culture, CBC, possible imaging, IV antibiotics, pain management adjustment. Collaborative: Notify surgeon, involve wound care if needed, pharmacy for antibiotic recommendations.

Exercise 5 — Take Action: Priority 1: Thorough wound assessment and vital signs. Priority 2: Notify surgeon/provider using SBAR—"I'm concerned Mrs. Patterson may be developing a surgical site infection. She has fever 101.2, WBC 13,200, uncontrolled pain, and her knee is warmer than expected." Priority 3: Implement orders when received, document thoroughly.

Exercise 6 — Evaluate Outcomes: Positive outcomes: Temperature normalizes, pain controlled, WBC decreasing, wound appearance improving. Warning signs: Increasing fever, spreading redness, purulent drainage, hemodynamic instability, altered mental status. Reassess: Every 2-4 hours until stable, after interventions.

Case Study 8.2 Answers — Emma (Pediatric Respiratory Distress)

Exercise 1 — Recognize Cues: Significant cues: Barking cough (pathognomonic for croup), inspiratory stridor at rest (indicates significant upper airway obstruction), moderate retractions and nasal flaring (increased work of breathing), SpO2 91% (hypoxia), HR 142 and RR 36 (compensatory responses), sudden nighttime onset after mild URI. Severity indicators: stridor at rest, retractions, hypoxia indicate moderate-severe croup.

Exercise 2 — Analyze Cues: Pattern: Upper airway obstruction from subglottic edema (croup/laryngotracheobronchitis). Albuterol didn't help because asthma affects lower airways (bronchospasm); croup affects upper airway (subglottic swelling). The obstruction is at the larynx/trachea level, hence the inspiratory stridor (air struggling to get IN through narrowed upper airway). No wheezing confirms this is not an asthma exacerbation.

Exercise 3 — Prioritize Hypotheses: Most likely: Croup (viral laryngotracheobronchitis)—classic presentation with barking cough, stridor, preceding URI, age group. Rule out: Epiglottitis (would see toxic appearance, drooling, tripod positioning, refusal to swallow, muffled voice—Emma is crying and consolable, which is reassuring). Also consider foreign body aspiration, though no choking history reported.

Exercise 4 — Generate Solutions: Medications: Dexamethasone (reduces airway edema—mainstay treatment), nebulized racemic epinephrine if severe (provides rapid temporary relief). Nursing comfort: Keep child calm (crying worsens stridor), allow to stay with parent, comfortable position (sitting on parent's lap). Environmental: Cool mist may help, avoid agitating the child.

Exercise 5 — Take Action: Immediate priorities: Apply oxygen, keep child calm with mother, administer dexamethasone. Communication with mother: "Emma has croup—it sounds scary but we can help her. The barking cough is from swelling in her airway. We're going to give medicine to reduce the swelling." AVOID:

Upsetting the child (worsens obstruction), separating from parent, examining throat if epiglottitis suspected (can cause complete obstruction).

Exercise 6 — Evaluate Outcomes: Improvement: Stridor resolving, decreased work of breathing, SpO2 improving, child calmer, able to drink fluids. Escalation needed: Worsening stridor, cyanosis, decreased level of consciousness, severe retractions, drooling (suggests epiglottitis). Discharge teaching: Croup often worsens at night, cool night air or steam may help, return if stridor at rest, difficulty breathing, or unable to drink.

Case Study 8.3 Answers — Mrs. Williams (Postpartum Hemorrhage)

Exercise 1 — Recognize Cues: Abnormal bleeding cues: Saturating 2 pads/hour (>1 pad/hour is excessive), heavy flow with clots, saturating pad in 30 minutes. Hemodynamic instability: Tachycardia 118, hypotension 94/58 (significant drop from baseline 118/72), lightheadedness, pale/cool/diaphoretic skin. Risk factors: Prolonged labor, Pitocin augmentation, large baby, multiparity.

Exercise 2 — Analyze Cues: Cause: Boggy fundus indicates uterine atony—the uterus is not contracting to compress bleeding vessels at placental site. Fundus above umbilicus suggests the uterus is filling with blood (uterine distension). Displaced to right indicates full bladder (bladder pushes uterus to the side and prevents proper contraction)—this is both a contributor and a finding.

Exercise 3 — Prioritize Hypotheses: Four T's: Tone (atony), Trauma (lacerations), Tissue (retained placenta), Thrombin (coagulation disorders). Most likely: Tone (uterine atony)—the boggy fundus directly indicates this. Must rule out: Retained placental fragments, cervical or vaginal lacerations (especially with prolonged pushing). If atony treatment doesn't work, consider trauma or tissue.

Exercise 4 — Generate Solutions: Immediate nursing: Fundal massage (stimulates contraction), have patient empty bladder (catheterize if needed—full bladder prevents uterine contraction). Medications: Oxytocin (Pitocin), methylergonovine (Methergine), carboprost (Hemabate), misoprostol. Bladder intervention addresses the displaced fundus.

Exercise 5 — Take Action: First action: Fundal massage while calling for help. Simultaneous: Call for help, catheterize bladder, start/increase IV, request uterotonics. Quantify blood loss by weighing pads and underpads (1 gram = 1 mL blood). This is an obstetric emergency—do not delay interventions.

Exercise 6 — Evaluate Outcomes: Improvement: Fundus becomes firm, bleeding decreases, vital signs stabilize. Escalation to OR/blood products: Fundus remains boggy despite massage and medications, continued heavy bleeding, vital signs worsening, estimated blood loss >1000mL. Ongoing monitoring: Vital signs q15min until stable, fundal checks, pad counts, I&O, H&H in 4-6 hours.

Case Study 8.4 Answers — Mr. Thomas (Suicide Risk Assessment)

Exercise 1 — Recognize Cues: Risk factors: Previous suicide attempt (strongest predictor), history of depression, recent near-lethal attempt (car in garage), presence of suicide note, medication non-compliance, job loss, social isolation, hopelessness. Warning signs: Statements of being a burden, wanting "pain to stop," flat affect, withdrawal. Protective factors: Cooperative with treatment, wife involved, accepting hospitalization.

Exercise 2 — Analyze Cues: Depression severity: Severe—hypersomnia (14-16 hours), significant weight loss, hopelessness, psychomotor retardation, functional impairment. Medication non-compliance increases risk because antidepressants take weeks to work; stopping abruptly can worsen depression and increase impulsivity. Suicide note indicates planning and intent—this was not an impulsive act.

Exercise 3 — Prioritize Hypotheses: Priority diagnosis: Risk for suicide related to recent attempt, major depression, and hopelessness. Suicide risk level: HIGH—recent near-lethal attempt, presence of note, multiple risk factors, severe depression, means access (was able to attempt), stated ambivalence about living. The passive death wish and ambivalence ("I don't know if I could do it again") does not reduce risk level.

Exercise 4 — Generate Solutions: Safety: 1:1 observation, remove all potential means (sharps, cords, etc.), safe environment. Therapeutic communication: Non-judgmental presence, active listening, validate feelings without reinforcing hopelessness, avoid platitudes. Medications: Restart antidepressant (may need different agent or dose), consider faster-acting adjuncts for acute phase.

Exercise 5 — Take Action: Observation: Continuous 1:1 observation (highest level) given recent near-lethal attempt. Safety measures: Room search, belongings check, sharps precautions, bathroom supervision. Building rapport: Consistent staff assignment, genuine interest without prying, availability, collaborative safety planning, validating his experience without reinforcing hopelessness.

Exercise 6 — Evaluate Outcomes: Decreased risk indicators: Engaging in treatment, future-oriented statements, improved affect, sleeping and eating better, developing coping strategies, verbalizing reasons for living. Increased risk indicators: Increased agitation, giving away possessions, sudden "calmness" after depression, secretive behavior, refusing to contract for safety. Discharge planning: Safety plan, means restriction at home, outpatient follow-up, family involvement, crisis resources.

Case Study 8.5 Answers — Mr. Jackson (Septic Shock)

Exercise 1 — Recognize Cues: Sepsis indicators: Fever 103.2°F, WBC 24,800, suspected source (UTI). Shock indicators: Hypotension 78/48 (MAP 58), tachycardia 128, tachypnea 28, altered mental status. Organ dysfunction: Renal (creatinine doubled from baseline), neurological (confusion), respiratory (hypoxia requiring supplemental O_2), metabolic (lactate 5.8 indicates tissue hypoperfusion).

Exercise 2 — Analyze Cues: Hemodynamic pattern: Distributive (septic) shock—vasodilation causes hypotension despite adequate volume. CVP elevated (12) after 2L fluid indicates he has volume but vessels are dilated and vasopressors are needed. Lactate 5.8 indicates severe tissue hypoperfusion—cells are in anaerobic metabolism. This is septic shock: sepsis + hypotension refractory to fluid + lactate >4.

Exercise 3 — Prioritize Hypotheses: Diagnosis: Septic shock secondary to urosepsis. Source evidence: UTI treated as outpatient (inadequate treatment), cloudy foul-smelling urine, elderly male (UTI common). Priority problems: (1) Shock/hypoperfusion, (2) Respiratory failure, (3) Acute kidney injury, (4) Altered mental status.

Exercise 4 — Generate Solutions: Sepsis bundle (Hour-1): Measure lactate, obtain blood cultures before antibiotics, administer broad-spectrum antibiotics, begin fluid resuscitation, apply vasopressors for MAP <65 after fluids. Hemodynamic support: Norepinephrine (first-line vasopressor for septic shock). Respiratory support: Likely needs intubation given hypoxia on 6L—prepare for rapid sequence intubation.

Exercise 5 — Take Action: Immediate priorities: (1) Establish arterial line and central access, (2) Start vasopressor, (3) Ensure broad-spectrum antibiotics infusing, (4) Prepare for intubation, (5) Place Foley for strict output monitoring. Monitoring: Continuous arterial BP, CVP trends, hourly lactate clearance, urine output, mental status. Family communication: This is critical illness, explain ICU level of care, likely intubation, serious but treatable if source controlled.

Exercise 6 — Evaluate Outcomes: Resuscitation targets: MAP ≥65, lactate decreasing (>10% per 2 hours), urine output ≥0.5 mL/kg/hr, improving mental status. Improvement signs: Decreasing vasopressor requirements, lactate clearing, improving oxygenation, urine output increasing. Refractory shock signs: Escalating vasopressor needs, worsening lactate, multi-organ failure progression, no response to source control—may need additional vasopressors, stress-dose steroids consideration.

Clinical Pearl: *In septic shock, time is critical. The Surviving Sepsis Campaign emphasizes that every hour of delay in antibiotic administration increases mortality. The Hour-1 bundle elements should be initiated immediately upon recognition, not after transfer or test results.*

10.10 Chapter 9 Answers — Comprehensive Practice Sets

Practice Set 9.1 Answers: Cardiac Emergency

9.1.1 — Recognize Cues: Select: Chest pressure radiating to left arm and jaw, Troponin I 0.08 ng/mL, Diaphoresis, Oxygen saturation 94%. Rationale: These are the findings requiring immediate attention as they indicate active myocardial ischemia/infarction. History items (HTN, smoking) and blood glucose are important but not requiring immediate attention.

9.1.2 — Analyze Cues: Chest pressure with radiation: Consistent. Elevated troponin: Consistent. Diaphoresis with anxiety: Consistent. Elevated blood glucose: Unrelated (may be stress response but not specific to ACS). Tachycardia: Consistent. Rationale: Classic ACS presentation includes chest discomfort with radiation, troponin elevation indicating myocardial damage, autonomic symptoms (diaphoresis), and compensatory tachycardia.

9.1.3 — Prioritize Hypotheses: DROPDOWN 1: NSTEMI. DROPDOWN 2: elevated troponin. DROPDOWN 3: cardiogenic shock. Rationale: Elevated troponin confirms myocardial injury (differentiates NSTEMI from unstable angina). Cardiogenic shock is the most dangerous complication—heart failure from damaged myocardium.

9.1.4 — Generate Solutions: Select: Administer aspirin 325 mg chewed, Apply supplemental oxygen, Obtain 12-lead ECG, Administer sublingual nitroglycerin, Start IV heparin infusion, Prepare for possible cardiac catheterization, Obtain serial troponins. NOT selected: Insulin (not priority for ACS management). Rationale: These interventions follow ACS protocols—antiplatelet therapy, oxygen for hypoxia, ECG for diagnosis/monitoring, nitrates for ischemia, anticoagulation, and cath lab preparation.

9.1.5 — Take Action: Order: 1-Obtain 12-lead ECG, 2-Apply oxygen, 3-Establish IV access, 4-Administer aspirin, 5-Administer nitroglycerin, 6-Notify cardiology. Rationale: ECG first to identify STEMI (changes management urgency). Oxygen for hypoxia. IV access enables medication administration. Aspirin immediately for antiplatelet effect. Nitro after access established. Cardiology after initial stabilization.

9.1.6 — Evaluate Outcomes: Pain 2/10: Improvement. BP 142/86: Improvement. Troponin 0.42: Deterioration (expected rise but indicates ongoing damage). No longer diaphoretic: Improvement. New crackles: Deterioration. Rationale: Troponin rise is expected but indicates infarct size. New crackles suggest developing pulmonary edema/heart failure—this is concerning and requires intervention.

Practice Set 9.2 Answers: Pediatric Infection

9.2.1 — Recognize Cues (Highlight): Highlight: T 103.8°F (high fever), HR 132 (tachycardia), dry mucous membranes, capillary refill 3 seconds (delayed), only one wet diaper (decreased output), lethargic. These indicate severity beyond simple ear infection—dehydration and systemic response to infection.

9.2.2 — Analyze Cues: Select for dehydration: Heart rate 132 (compensatory), Dry mucous membranes, Capillary refill 3 seconds, Only one wet diaper, Decreased activity. NOT dehydration indicators: Temperature (infection sign), Bulging TMs (local infection sign). Rationale: Tachycardia compensates for decreased volume, mucous membranes and capillary refill indicate perfusion, decreased urine output is key dehydration marker.

9.2.3 — Prioritize Hypotheses: DROPDOWN 1: acute otitis media. DROPDOWN 2: mild dehydration. DROPDOWN 3: fluid resuscitation (or treating the ear infection—both acceptable). DROPDOWN 4:

dehydration can progress to shock. Rationale: Bilateral bulging TMs confirm AOM. Dehydration signs present but not severe. Both rehydration and infection treatment are priorities.

9.2.4 — Generate Solutions: Select: Oral rehydration solution, Acetaminophen, Amoxicillin, Warm compress, Follow-up in 48-72 hours. NOT selected: Immediate IV bolus (mild dehydration—oral rehydration appropriate), Hospitalization (not indicated for uncomplicated AOM with mild dehydration), Lumbar puncture (no meningitis signs—alert, consolable, no neck stiffness).

9.2.5 — Take Action: Priority order: 1-Signs of worsening infection (safety/return precautions first), 2-Fever and pain management (immediate comfort), 3-Pushing fluids (ongoing hydration), 4-Importance of completing antibiotics (treatment adherence), 5-When to return for follow-up. Rationale: Parents must know danger signs first. Comfort measures enable the child to drink and recover.

9.2.6 — Evaluate Outcomes: Temp 100.2°F: Treatment working. 4 wet diapers: Treatment working. Still pulling at ears: Monitor (pain may persist 24-48 hrs). Eating half breakfast: Treatment working. Rash after antibiotic: Immediate evaluation. Rationale: Fever trending down and improved urine output are positive. Rash could indicate allergic reaction—needs immediate assessment to determine if drug allergy vs. viral exanthem.

Practice Set 9.3 Answers: Obstetric Emergency

9.3.1 — Recognize Cues: Select ALL of these for severe features: BP 172/110 (severe range ≥160/110), Severe headache, Visual disturbances, Elevated liver enzymes, Thrombocytopenia, Hyperreflexia with clonus, Proteinuria. NOT severe feature: Gestational age 34 weeks (timing, not severity), FHR 145 with moderate variability (reassuring, not pathological).

9.3.2 — Analyze Cues: Headache/visual changes: Neurological. Elevated AST/ALT: Hepatic. Platelets 98,000: Hematologic. Proteinuria/creatinine: Renal. Hyperreflexia/clonus: Neurological. Rationale: Preeclampsia is a multi-system disease affecting brain (cerebral edema), liver, platelets (consumption), kidneys, and causing CNS hyperexcitability that can lead to seizures.

9.3.3 — Prioritize Hypotheses: DROPDOWN 1: preeclampsia with severe features. DROPDOWN 2: maternal seizure (eclampsia). DROPDOWN 3: delivery of the baby. Rationale: Multiple severe features present. Headache, visual changes, and hyperreflexia/clonus indicate imminent seizure risk. Delivery removes the placenta—the source of the pathology.

9.3.4 — Generate Solutions: Select: Magnesium sulfate (seizure prophylaxis), IV antihypertensive (labetalol/hydralazine), Betamethasone (fetal lungs at 34 weeks), Continuous fetal monitoring, Foley catheter (monitor output/mag toxicity), Seizure precautions, Preparation for delivery. NOT: Bed rest at home (severe preeclampsia requires hospitalization and likely delivery).

9.3.5 — Take Action: Order: 1-Initiate continuous fetal monitoring (assess fetal status), 2-Administer magnesium sulfate (seizure prevention is priority), 3-Administer IV antihypertensive (prevent stroke), 4-Draw labs, 5-Insert Foley catheter, 6-Notify neonatology. Rationale: Fetal assessment and seizure prevention are highest priorities. BP control prevents maternal stroke.

9.3.6 — Evaluate Outcomes: BP 148/92: Desired outcome (improvement from 172/110). DTRs 2+: Desired outcome (clonus resolved). Urine output 15 mL/hr: Complication (oliguria—could indicate worsening disease or magnesium toxicity). RR 10, drowsy: Complication (magnesium toxicity signs—hold mag, check level, have calcium gluconate ready). FHR 140, moderate variability: Desired outcome (reassuring fetal status).

Practice Set 9.4 Answers: Mental Health Crisis

9.4.1 — Recognize Cues: Select for manic episode: Not sleeping 4 days (decreased need for sleep), Rapid pressured speech, Grandiose beliefs, Reckless financial behavior, Irritability, Easily distracted, Risky behavior. Supporting but not diagnostic: Previous depressive episode (suggests bipolar), Family history, Elevated HR (physiological response to activity/agitation).

9.4.2 — Analyze Cues: DROPDOWN 1: manic episode. DROPDOWN 2: bipolar I disorder. DROPDOWN 3: harm from impaired judgment. Rationale: Full manic episode (not hypomania—impairment is significant). Bipolar I = depression + mania (Bipolar II = depression + hypomania only). She's engaging in dangerous behavior (directing traffic) due to impaired judgment.

9.4.3 — Prioritize Hypotheses: Safety risk from impaired judgment: High. Physical effects of sleep deprivation: High. Ruling out medical causes: High. Risk of progression to psychosis: Moderate. Financial consequences: Low (important but not immediate clinical priority). Rationale: Safety is always first. Sleep deprivation and medical causes must be addressed. Grandiosity can progress to psychotic delusions.

9.4.4 — Generate Solutions: Select: Psychiatric admission, Mood stabilizer, Antipsychotic, Benzodiazepine, Low-stimulation environment, Medical workup. NOT selected: SSRI (can trigger/worsen mania), Encouraging business plans (reinforces grandiosity, not therapeutic). Rationale: She needs stabilization. Mood stabilizers are mainstay treatment. Antipsychotics and benzos help acute symptoms. Rule out thyroid disease and substances.

9.4.5 — Take Action: Order: 1-Ensure safe environment (always first), 2-Establish therapeutic rapport (enables all other interventions), 3-Complete medical clearance labs (rule out medical causes), 4-Set firm consistent limits (manage behavior), 5-Administer PRN medication (if needed for agitation), 6-Contact family (collateral information). Rationale: Safety and rapport foundation. Medical workup before psychiatric treatment. Limits before sedation if possible.

9.4.6 — Evaluate Outcomes: Sleeping 5 hours: Improvement (was 0). Speech slowing: Improvement. Still believes idea is brilliant: No change (grandiosity may take longer to resolve). Less irritable: Improvement. Tremor: Concern (could be lithium side effect—check level, assess for toxicity). Rationale: Sleep improvement is key early sign of treatment response. Tremor requires evaluation—lithium therapeutic window is narrow.

Practice Set 9.5 Answers: Respiratory Failure

9.5.1 — Recognize Cues: Select for respiratory failure: SpO_2 84%, $PaCO_2$ 58, pH 7.31, Using accessory muscles, Speaking in 2-3 word sentences, RR 32. NOT specific to respiratory failure: Temperature (indicates infection cause), History of COPD (background, not acute finding). Rationale: Hypoxemia, hypercapnia, acidosis, and clinical signs of respiratory distress define respiratory failure.

9.5.2 — Analyze Cues: DROPDOWN 1: respiratory acidosis. DROPDOWN 2: partially compensated. DROPDOWN 3: chronic CO_2 retention. DROPDOWN 4: hypercapnic (Type 2). Rationale: Low pH + high CO_2 = respiratory acidosis. Elevated HCO_3 (28) indicates kidneys have been compensating (chronic). Type 2 respiratory failure = hypercapnia (CO_2 retention); Type 1 = hypoxemia only.

9.5.3 — Prioritize Hypotheses: COPD exacerbation from viral infection: Most likely (URI prodrome, classic presentation). Bacterial pneumonia: Possible (fever, productive cough—may be superinfection). PE: Possible (always consider in acute dyspnea). Heart failure: Possible (can coexist/exacerbate COPD). Pneumothorax: Unlikely (no pleuritic pain, breath sounds diminished but not absent).

9.5.4 — Generate Solutions: Select: Titrate oxygen to 88-92% (NOT >94%—CO_2 retainer), Nebulized bronchodilators, Systemic corticosteroids, Antibiotics, BiPAP, Chest X-ray. NOT selected: Oxygen >94% (suppresses hypoxic drive in COPD), Immediate intubation (try BiPAP first unless severe distress/altered consciousness). Rationale: COPD patients rely on hypoxic drive; over-oxygenation worsens CO_2 retention. BiPAP can prevent intubation.

9.5.5 — Take Action: Order: 1-Apply controlled oxygen therapy (address hypoxia safely), 2-Administer nebulized bronchodilators (open airways), 3-Initiate BiPAP (support ventilation), 4-Administer IV corticosteroids (reduce inflammation), 5-Obtain chest X-ray (identify cause), 6-Start antibiotics (treat presumed infection). Rationale: Oxygenation first but controlled. Bronchodilation for immediate relief. BiPAP to reduce work of breathing and improve CO2 clearance.

9.5.6 — Evaluate Outcomes: ABG improving (pH 7.35, CO2 down, PO2 up): Improvement. RR 24, less accessory muscle use: Improvement. Speaking full sentences: Improvement. Drowsy, difficult to arouse: Deterioration (CO2 narcosis or fatigue—may need intubation). SpO2 91%: Improvement (in target range for COPD). Rationale: ABG and clinical signs improving, but altered mental status is ominous—indicates possible ventilatory failure despite BiPAP. Prepare for intubation.

Clinical Pearl: *In COPD patients, a drowsy or somnolent patient despite treatment is an ominous sign of CO2 narcosis and impending respiratory arrest. Do not delay intubation if mental status declines even if other parameters are improving.*

References

Alfaro-LeFevre, R. (2020). *Critical thinking, clinical reasoning, and clinical judgment: A practical approach* (7th ed.). Elsevier.

Benner, P. (1984). *From novice to expert: Excellence and power in clinical nursing practice.* Addison-Wesley.

Dickison, P., Haerling, K. A., & Lasater, K. (2019). Integrating the National Council of State Boards of Nursing Clinical Judgment Model into nursing educational frameworks. *Journal of Nursing Education, 58*(2), 72-78. https://doi.org/10.3928/01484834-20190122-03

Institute for Healthcare Improvement. (2021). *SBAR tool: Situation-Background-Assessment-Recommendation.* http://www.ihi.org/resources/Pages/Tools/SBARToolkit.aspx

Jones, D. A., DeVita, M. A., & Bellomo, R. (2013). Rapid-response teams. *New England Journal of Medicine, 365*(2), 139-146. https://doi.org/10.1056/NEJMra0910926

Melnyk, B. M., & Fineout-Overholt, E. (2019). *Evidence-based practice in nursing and healthcare: A guide to best practice* (4th ed.). Wolters Kluwer.

National Council of State Boards of Nursing. (2016). *National guidelines for nursing delegation.* https://www.ncsbn.org/NGND-PosePaper_06.pdf

National Council of State Boards of Nursing. (2018). *NCSBN Clinical Judgment Measurement Model.* https://www.ncsbn.org/public-files/Measuring_Clinical_Judgment_NCSBN.pdf

National Council of State Boards of Nursing. (2023). *Next Generation NCLEX (NGN) resources.* https://www.ncsbn.org/next-generation-nclex.htm

Tanner, C. A. (2006). Thinking like a nurse: A research-based model of clinical judgment in nursing. *Journal of Nursing Education, 45*(6), 204-211.

Made in United States
Orlando, FL
04 November 2026

90201054R00070